Massage cures

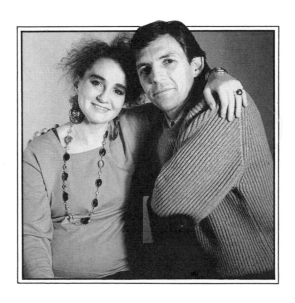

MASSAGE CURES

The family guide to curing common ailments with simple massage
techniques

Nigel Dawes and Fiona Harrold

THORSONS PUBLISHING GROUP

First published in 1990

British Library Cataloguing in Publication Data

Dawes, Nigel
Massage cures.
1. Man. Therapy. Massage
I. Title II. Harrold, Fiona
615.822

ISBN 0 7225 2180 4

Published by Thorsons Publishers Limited, Wellingborough, Northamptonshire, NN8 2RQ, England

Printed in Great Britain by B.L.&U., Wellingborough, Northamptonshire
Typesetting by MJL Limited, Hitchin, Hertfordshire

1 3 5 7 9 10 8 6 4 2

Contents

Acknowledgements

The authors wish to thank Felicity and Andrew for their constant love and support throughout the writing of this book, and always.

Special thanks also to the following for their contribution to the book:

Mark and Jeff
Rachel
Klara-Gaia
Barbara
Robin
Amanda and Chris
Vip and Jo

Shion
Galia and Jade
Lavinia and Rosamond
Simone and Phil
Margaret
Tony and Norma Dawes
Catherine

Introduction -
the power of touch

Touch is a fundamental human instinct and need. Human culture has consistently used touch as a means for communication, whether in a therapeutic context or simply as an expression of care and affection. There is little doubt that structured touching has been around for as long as the human race itself.

In our language, we as humans clearly appreciate the role of touch. We describe the quality and closeness of our relationships in terms of 'being in touch' or 'out of touch'. We talk of being 'touched', 'deeply touched' when describing our reaction to something or someone who has impressed us in a certain way, and of not wanting to 'touch' something that we are unsure about. The importance of skin is also reflected in our speech: we speak of 'thick-skinned' people and those who are 'tactful' or 'tactless', 'unfeeling' or 'callous'.

For some so-called primitive cultures, close touch is a way of life: for example, babies are held or carried by working mothers and later by their older brothers and sisters. This can be seen in such diverse cultures as the Eskimos and the bushmen of Borneo which each display their own individual but uniform use of touch in their societies as a basis of identification, communication and growth.

This phenomenon can also be seen very clearly in the animal kingdom where touch plays a crucial role in the creation, birth and rearing of offspring. Animals instinctively lick their offspring and there are societies where this practice is common among humans, such as in Tibet and among the Polar Eskimos. It is even possible that the 'licking' of humans is provided by the long labour period during birth, but it is certain that the newborn human is thoroughly immature and totally dependent on its mother to a far greater degree than any other infant in the animal kingdom, with the exception of the ape family.

Throughout our life and especially in early postnatal stages we are therefore in a rapid state of growth and development, a large part of which depends on touch. In fact, a condition known as *marasmus* has been identified whereby newborn babies that are deprived of touch actually waste away and die. Animal research has shown that caressing and tender touch in early life accelerates the natural development of the whole organism, stimulating skeletal and body growth, improving digestion and assimilation, and stimulating the hormone system. This may account for the positive effect of massage on stress and the immune system.

Touch also strongly affects the autonomic nervous system, simultaneously relaxing and energizing the body, and research has shown that it encourages the release of endorphines, known as 'happy hormones', which act as the body's natural opiates in reducing pain and producing a feeling of elation and well-being.

Whole person therapy

Touch also has a clear role to play in the psychological and behavioural development of the whole person. Modern psychology is only just beginning to research and establish clear, defined links between early parent-child bonding patterns, primarily established through touch, and patterns of behaviour in later life. Unfortunately, the overwhelming influence of Freud in the practice of modern psychiatry has meant that touch during therapy has been considered taboo. It was only through the work of Wilhelm Reich and others like him that the idea of treating the mind *and* body together started to gain ground. The fact that all the 'hands on' therapies practised today have a clear framework for treating the mind and body is an obvious indication of the need for whole person therapy.

We do not generally regard the skin as an organ, but in fact, next to the brain, the skin is the most important of all our organ systems and certainly the most sensitive. Its very early development in prenatal life points to its fundamental importance to the organism. The sense most closely associated with it is touch and is our first medium of communication since it is through our skin that we can literally 'keep in touch' with our immediate environment. It acts in effect as an external nervous system keeping us informed about what is going on around us, regulating temperature and metabolism and protecting us against injury or invasion from the outside.

Our senses develop in a well-defined sequence: tactile, auditory and visual and this distinguishes touch as the most significant influence on our early development. The loss or absence of other senses is never life-threatening, unlike the condition *Cutaneous Analgia* where the affected person experiences no pain on the skin and may easily inflict serious injury on him- or herself without realizing. In fact, the ability of people such as Helen Keller to interpret the richness and colour of their world came through their touch. The Braille alphabet allows blind people to communicate through touch.

In the Far East, massage became the traditional domain of blind people whose sense of touch was so accentuated and subtly refined. Indeed in massage today, we talk of 'tuning into' the body with our hands and 'switching off' the other senses. Many doctors will still lay a hand on their patients in initial consultation today to elicit information about the patient's condition simply through touch.

The interesting point about touch and massage is that it is already done on an unconscious level which is well expressed in the mother-child relationship, where a mother will instinctively rub her child's pain away simply by holding the sore part, or console a crying baby through hugging and stroking. However, it is not merely touch that heals and comforts, but a certain quality in the touch. We have all witnessed a child being held in a way where care was not necessarily being conveyed, but perhaps intense irritation. This communication has quite the opposite result.

At the post-infant stage, touch comes naturally into the daily life of a child through play, an element of life which is all too easily forgotten by the adult. Even sickness, on one level, can be seen as an attention-seeker, often disguising a desperate need to be touched. Interestingly, where touch is missing in our lives, it invariably finds some way to express itself whether at sports matches, in greeting one another or when we actively seek it in the form of a massage. Sadly, this essential desire for touch is often suppressed and may find distorted and potentially harmful ways of expressing itself which may include violent or sexually abusive behaviour.

The currently much-discussed issue of child abuse is a clear example of this. The danger is that parents may overreact to this situation by withholding natural physical contact for fear of their behaviour being misinterpreted. This is a vicious circle which actually feeds the suppression of our instinctive desire to express our love and care through touch.

The message of touch

Clearly, then, we can convey precise messages to another human being through our touch. The touch may look the same, but on different occasions can convey distinctly different messages and therefore elicit different responses as a consequence. When we hold someone's hand or put our arm around them to offer reassurance we are letting them know that they are not alone, we are on their side and we can be counted on for support. This message conveyed through touch is much more powerful than the spoken word. Touch bonds us to another human being in a way that leaves us with a profound sense of reassurance and 'connectedness'.

Touch is a way of communication that goes beyond words in a way that words can never adequately capture. Indeed, it may be that we have to invent a new language to speak of how caring touch affects us. People will often fumble for the words and will speak of 'feeling balanced', 'at peace with themselves' or 'back to centre'. The recipient of a caring message will feel that their body is 'purring' with pleasure and contentment.

Unfortunately, we in the West do not welcome touch in our culture in the way that others do, or as we used to. In the United Kingdom, particularly, there is a distinct touch taboo and scientific research informs us that people in Britain touch less than in any other country! This situation can be traced back to clear historical trends: in the Middle Ages the Christian world held contempt for the body and 'worldly pleasures' in general, and massage suffered as a result. Massage has never completely recovered from this, and in this century became associated with prostitution. This has resulted in the simplistic connection of touch with sexual intimacy with no room for any other behaviour in between! Indeed, for many people the very word massage conjures up a rather unwholesome image. Perhaps most of all it was the Victorian era in Britain which really affected our attitudes towards touch, its constricting clothing symbolizing the repressive morality lurking beneath.

For many people their experience of touch is intrusive and unwelcome. This is painfully true for the city commuter who visibly shrinks from any contact with the other occupants of a crowded carriage on the train. It is also socially appropriate to apologize for any accidental contact made. In fact large overcrowded cities do restrict our physical space and we become guarded and threatened by our lack of choice in being touched.

First impressions

This lack of welcome caring touch can be traced back to birth. Modern birth practices have largely neglected the crucial bonding relationship between mother and newborn baby. As a baby our only relationship with the world was through touch. From touch we learned clear messages about how welcome we were, how loved and wanted we were and how important we were. In essence our self-worth was shaped forever through touch in those first days of life. It may well be that our whole future and sense of identity and our relationship with the world and other people is sculpted by this primary contact. First impressions last forever.

For those who did not experience adequate loving touch, caring massage may be the key to feeling more loved and supported by others. When we feel cared for and appreciated, we feel better about ourselves and this has immediate and wide-ranging ramifications. Through feeling more supported we open up and allow more fun and lightness and closeness with others into our lives.

The touch that we do experience as young children tends to reduce around the age of seven years. This is particularly true for boys as it is the age when sleeping with mother or parent is deemed to be no longer appropriate. This worsens with the onset of puberty, when physical contact may be reduced to an absolute minimum at a time when the reassurance of touch is most valuable. Aspects of our education system compound this process, and in many schools touch is more often associated with negative experiences like corporal punishment, bullying and peer group fighting. A strong case could be made in fact for a lack of touch or abusive touch being responsible for wide-ranging problems in later life which may include various addictions, violence and abusive behaviour, mental disease, and many so-called 'anti-social' conditions.

Recent research into the treatment of cancer and AIDS has shown that a caring hand is an essential part of the healing process. In areas of modern medicine where traditionally drugs are the only form of treatment, notably in psychiatry and geriatrics, touch may be the only way that people can retain a sense of dignity and self-worth.

Stress and tension

Stress and tension are now a part of everyday life for many people. Coping with a demanding job, a busy social and family life can all take their toll. This can take the shape of everyday ailments such as tiredness, fatigue, stiffness and tension, aches and pains which we all learn to put up with over time. This leads to a gradual and insidious running down of our general level of health and the state of our body eventually leading to illness, disease and premature ageing. Stress and busy lifestyle are not in themselves bad for us; however, how we react and deal with them is what can damage our health.

The progress of modern society has been so rapid and so revolutionary in all areas of life that we have now created an environment to which we must adequately respond in order to survive. History has taught us that adapting to changes in our environment on all levels is crucial to our survival as a species. The dinosaurs were unable to make this transition and consequently died out.

We have seen how, as humans, our primary response to our environment is our complex lifestyle, but to cope with this and its attendant stresses adequately, more and more people are returning to simple, natural means of preserving our health through touch. In an increasingly volatile world, people are literally 'reaching out', perhaps to regain the sense of communication and peace of mind experienced in earlier life. The thought of 'growing old alone' is what terrifies most and it may be that, through touch, whether in a structured, professional way as in massage, or just holding hands and hugging, we may stimulate our minds and bodies towards increasing vigour and zest.

History

The history of massage is well documented and probably dates from 3000 BC. The Indian books of the Ayur Veda, written about 1800 BC, refer to massage as a therapeutic healing art whilst wall paintings of foot massage (now known as reflexology) are a well-known feature of Egyptian culture. In China the oldest recorded medical treatise, the *Nei Ching*, written more than 1000 BC by the legendary 'Yellow Emperor', records in detail the classical theory and practice of Oriental medicine and includes many references to the art of massage. In it the different treatment forms of Chinese medicine including acupuncture, moxibustion, herbs and massage are said to have originated according to the various illnesses experienced by the peoples of different regions, each with their distinct climate, food and lifestyle. The people of the central region, for example, 'eat mixed food and do not [suffer or weary at their] toil'. They are described as suffering from 'complete paralysis, chills and fever' and 'are most fittingly treated with. . . massage of the skin and flesh. . . .' This description suggests that massage was chosen to treat people who led sedentary lives and suffered from circulatory, neurological and musculo-skeletal problems. This ties in with the modern practice of massage and its present-day relevance.

There is much documented evidence of the practice and benefits of massage in ancient Greek and Roman cultures. Socrates and Plato both praised massage in their writings whilst Herodicus affirmed that massage could cure disease and preserve health. His most famous pupil, Hippocrates, was perhaps the most famous champion of massage and his work the *Corpus Hippocraticum*, roughly contemporary to the *Nei Ching*, detailed the ethical and practical duties of a doctor amongst which the laying on of hands and the practice of massage were deemed essential. In ancient Rome Julius Caesar had daily massage for his neuralgia and Pliny had massage for his asthma.

Massage, or at least the laying on of hands and palm healing, is mentioned in almost all the major world religions, and the Bible is full of such references. In temples and monasteries, especially in the East, massage was considered an essential skill.

In the Middle Ages however, the Christian world held contempt for the body and 'worldly pleasures' in general and massage suffered as a result, only to reappear after the Renaissance. Much of the knowledge of the ancient massage traditions of China, Japan, Egypt, India, Greece and Rome was then rediscovered. Great golden age physicians like Ambroise Paré and Mercurialis revived interest in the subject and established its credentials amongst the medical community.

Per Henrik Ling, a native of Sweden, was the first to introduce massage systematically into Europe where it became known as 'Swedish Massage'. Currently all forms of massage are undergoing radical transformation in the West, both in terms of treatment and for relaxation. The medical profession is beginning to take a clear interest in the natural, well-proven therapeutic value of a medical system as old as the human race itself. Shiatsu, reflexology, aromatherapy, acupressure and massage as well as chiropractic and osteopathy are all flourishing today as a result of renewed interest in natural, preventative healthcare.

Prevention rather than cure

This trend reflects our growing awareness of the need to assume a measure of responsibility in looking after our health. Prevention rather than cure seems to be a prime motivating force behind many present-day pursuits like aerobic exercise, keep-fit, the martial arts, special diets and meditation, as well as the many therapies which deal with preventative measures for health. In the *Nei Ching* it states 'the superior physician helps before the early budding of the disease'; indeed surgery, often performed in ancient China, was looked down on as a last resort in treatment resulting from inferior medical practice. Traditionally, people would pay their doctors for keeping them in good health and not for treating them in sickness. The *Nei Ching* goes on to suggest that 'those who treat should be free from illness'.

Today, people are increasingly looking to be inspired towards greater health by contributing substantially to this process themselves and by getting support from health professionals whose own health is beyond question. It seems ironic perhaps that modern doctors still swear allegiance to the Hippocratic doctrine, almost all of which, save its ethical principles, is completely outmoded in terms of current medical practice. Its contemporary the *Nei Ching*, however, is still a standard textbook for all medical students in China and has lost none of its authority in the classical practice of Oriental medicine. Of course, it was not written as a mere textbook of medicine but rather as a treatise on the entire philosophy of health and disease.

It is perhaps the wider perspective on the nature of health and the whole person that we are rediscovering today. Increasingly, people are seeking to balance quality with quantity in their lives. They seek a long, fulfilled and totally happy life, free from illness and disease. Once again we may learn a great deal from the ancient Oriental philosophy of life in which longevity and health were considered identical. The very process of ageing itself was considered a sign of disease and those wishing to remain healthy and forever youthful and vital merely had to follow and obey the laws of nature.

Talking of the ancient sages the *Nei Ching* says 'they were tranquilly content in nothingness and the true vital force accompanied them always. Their vital spirit was preserved within. How then could illness come to them?' If we could distil all the ancient wisdom of different cultures it may simply boil down to living without stress in health and happiness with our fellow humans. As the French say, 'être bien dans sa peau' is our simplest ambition. Interestingly, the image used in this expression equating to our 'peace of mind' is one of feeling literally 'at home in one's skin'.

It is through creating this sense of inner peace and harmony within ourselves that we contribute to the peace of our environment, and make a difference in the world at large.

1

Massage therapies - a summary

Massage is a formalized system of touch which makes use of the innate ability and desire to touch that we all have. The various systems of massage give us access to the precise therapeutic function of touch. Massage has the potential to relax mind and body, or invigorate and stimulate. It is an unparalleled method for treating many diverse complaints and conditions. It treats and impacts the whole person, which makes it valuable in the treatment of all illness regardless of specific symptoms.

Massage is an ancient healing art which is now recognized as an extraordinary method of treatment for all modern 20th-century diseases. It is valuable in the treatment of all the effects of prolonged stress, such as heart and circulatory disorders; high blood pressure; mental and physical tension; lethargy; insomnia, and hyperactivity. It is the supreme balancer, bringing peace to a troubled mind and relief to a tense body.

However, massage goes beyond the relief of stress and pain. It works on and affects our overall well-being, our spirit. We may feel a deep sense of peace and contentment within ourselves, such as we have never felt before. We may feel in touch with a deeper part of ourselves, an inner voice. Massage can often be the key to opening a spiritual perspective or dimension to our lives.

The most familiar types of massage today are Swedish massage and holistic (intuitive) massage. Swedish massage involves a set series of strokes designed to provoke specific physiological effects in the body. Holistic or intuitive massage has grown and developed since the 1960s, based on this basic framework. As the name suggests, it takes into account the whole person, mentally and emotionally as well as physically. This difference manifests mainly in holding the perspective that massage affects the whole person. On a practical level it means we are discerning about the types of strokes used and the speed of the strokes. Emphasis is placed on quality of touch above all else. It is just as important to have a clear intention and caring attitude as it is to perform the strokes and techniques in the correct way. Within the context of this, back massage techniques, both Eastern and Western, will be outlined as a first aid treatment, as a preventative treatment, and as a tool to enhance overall health and happiness.

Oriental massage and medical theory have a perspective on energy which we do not have in the West. This perspective allows us to think of having energy in the body either to be strengthened or released, depending on whether it is deficient or excessive. This energy called *Ki*, or *cho*, or *prana* is also thought to be directly connected to the internal organs of the body. This outlook is reflected in acupuncture, acupressure and shiatsu, the most popular systems of Oriental massage.

Aromatherapy

Aromatherapy is the use of essential oils for the treatment of mind and body. Essential oils are the 'life-force', the essence of the plants, flowers, fruits and trees from which they are extracted. They have a powerful effect on the human body and can provide benefits for a wide range of health problems from aches and pains to digestive problems and skin complaints. The use of plants and their oils has been practised for thousands of years, probably originating in China before moving via India to the Middle East.

In this century a French chemist, René-Maurice Gattefosse, and a doctor, Jean Valnet, rediscovered the healing properties of oils. Valnet used essential oils to treat injuries during World War I and his book is still available. Valnet's work was carried on by Marguerite Maury, an Austrian biochemist, who pioneered the modern approach to aromatheraphy. She developed a style of treatment which relied on massage for the application of the oils. She found this combination created an energy capable of relaxing or stimulating both mind and body, enhancing the body's natural healing ability and generally contributing to good health and wellbeing. Modern aromatherapy is alive and flourishing and its potential is being newly researched and rediscovered.

In this book you will find oils being recommended to be used in massage, baths or handkerchief inhalation, or as compresses. Below is outlined the descriptions of these methods.

Massage: The essential oils are carried through the skin in a vegetable oil in a ration of one drop of essential oil to 2ml of vegetable oil. A whole body treatment will normally require 25ml vegetable oil with 12 drops essential oil. A back will require 10ml with 5 drops of essential oil.

Steam Inhalation: To a bowl of steaming water, add 5 to 10 drops of essential oil. Then place a towel over your head and the bowl and inhale the vapour for a few minutes. This can be repeated two or three times a day.

Handkerchief Inhalations: Apply three or four drops of the essential oil to a handkerchief and inhale as often as you feel the need.

Baths: Fill the bath with water and add 5 to 10 drops to the water. Agitate and mix well. For a relaxing bath allow yourself at least 15 minutes to soak in the benefits.

Compresses: Compresses can be either cold or hot. Add 10 drops to 100ml of water. Soak a piece of cotton wool or soft towel and place on the area. To keep the compress hot, place a plastic bag over it and hold a hot water bottle on it.

Caution — The oils must never be taken internally, unless prescribed by a qualified and experienced aromatherapist. Never use the oils without first diluting them in the vegetable oil. Do not use larger amounts than recommended. Do not use the source oil daily for longer than three weeks or it may build up in your system and become toxic. Oils to be avoided during pregnancy are: Arnica, Basil, Clary Sage, Cypress, Fennel, Frankincense, Hyssop, Jasmine, Juniper, Marjoram, Myrrh, Pennyroyal, Peppermint, Rosemary, Sage, Thyme and Wintergreen. Essential oils should be used with extra caution for children. Always dilute essential oils before adding them to the bath and never use more than 4 drops. Use half the amount of oils in a massage mixture of that you would use for adults.

Finally do not attempt to treat a serious illness with aromatherapy alone. The oils will support a holistic programme of treatment or any orthodox medical treatment you or your partner or friend may be undergoing.

Shiatsu

Shiatsu is a form of Oriental massage which, like acupuncture, aims to stimulate and balance the body's own energy. It involves pressure, applied with hands, knees, elbows and feet to energy lines, *meridians*, all over the body. The result is to release areas of tension and strengthen areas of weakness, improving circulation and flexibility to give a strong sense of vitality as well as deep feeling of relaxation and wellbeing. The word Shiatsu means literally 'finger pressure' and distinguishes a therapeutic discipline incorporating elements of traditional massage as well as more recent techniques including physiotherapy and osteopathy/chiropractic. It employs the same fundamental diagnostic and treatment principles as the other Oriental medical practices of acupuncture, moxibustion and herbal medicine and is mentioned together with these disciplines in the first recorded medical classic, the *Nei Ching Su Wen*, written almost 3000 years ago. Today Shiatsu is growing in popularity in the West and is increasingly being seen as an effective way of staying healthy and enhancing vitality as well as for the treatment of common ailments.

Bach flower remedies

These are essences prepared from the flowers of wild plants, bushes and trees. They were developed by an eminent Harley Street consultant and bacteriologist, Dr Edward Bach, in the 1930s. Dr Bach had become disillusioned with the constant treating of symptoms with medicines which often had harmful side-effects. He came to the understanding that every physical symptom has an underlying root cause, stemming from a mental or emotional problem. He concluded that the only way to convert the disorder was to treat not merely the symptom, but the root cause as well. He characterized 38 negative mental and emotional states that we are all prone to, and developed a remedy for each state. The remedies work to alleviate states of mental or emotional anguish which would otherwise block the free flowing of the person's life-force, resulting in physical illness.

Directions

The remedies can be taken individually or in a combination of up to three. They can safely be taken internally (a few drops in a glass of spring water four times a day), or almost fill a 30ml dropper bottle with spring water and add two drops of the chosen remedy or combinations. The remedies are not addictive, nor do they have any harmful side-effects. They can be safely given to children, plants and animals. With animals, add a few drops of the concentrate to their food, or rub in behind their ears.

Self-esteem

Self-esteem is healthy! It is about accepting and appreciating yourself, being a good friend to yourself, and treating yourself well. It is about enjoying inner contentment and peace of mind with a quiet reassurance and respect for your self-worth as a human being. Self-esteem is not about being arrogant, selfish or tyrannical towards others. It is only when we have neglected ourselves and are desperately needy that we behave in an inconsiderate, anti-social way.

A great deal of stress and anxiety is generated out of a deep-rooted lack of confidence in ourselves. Many of us live in perpetual fear that we won't be good enough or that we aren't good enough. But we've managed to do a good covering-up job all along! We may have gone through life feeling we'd got by through cheating, or convincing others that we were up to the mark when in fact we weren't. This sets up a dangerous cycle where we are always compensating for our inherent lack by striving to prove our worth and value. The recognition this struggle brings is only temporary, for our true selves could merely be shown up at any time. And the more convincing our act, the more guilty we are likely to feel at misleading everyone.

There are ways out of this damaging and dangerous cycle. Firstly, it may come as an incredible surprise to know that the vast majority of the population shares your secret! Most people operate from the belief that 'I'm not good enough' and go to great lengths to hide this thought from themselves and everyone else. What a relief to know that everyone you know probably believes this about themselves! So it is very important to realize that this personal feature is actually a very common human trait. Its particular place of origin is personal to you, but the fact that the majority of people share its conclusion makes it an almost universal human trait. The thoughts and beliefs we hold about ourselves actually have a real effect in our world. They shape how we see and feel about ourselves, how we plan and imagine our life will be, and also how other people see us and treat us.

The most obvious example of this is at an important interview. Our thoughts may be 'not good enough . . . not really for this job . . . not up to it' and so on. Our interviewer will pick up on our discomfort and unease; in fact, without knowing it we greatly influence the overall impression we give. Therefore, it is extremely important to begin to train ourselves to be aware of the thoughts that we hold about ourselves and give expression to.

Thankfully, there are tried-and-tested ways of minimizing the effects of self-destructive thinking. The most important step is to notice immediately when we begin to indulge in damaging thoughts; as from this moment we are no longer at the mercy of them or controlled by them.

The next step is to acknowledge that they are only thoughts and are not 'real' unless we give them permission to be. We may have ample evidence from our past and childhood that they are true, but this has only been because we nurtured limitation around ourselves. Thankfully, we no longer need to do this and we can let go of the limiting thoughts as they come into our awareness.

Finally, we can actively replace negative thoughts with more affirming ones. This is simply choosing to believe different, more supportive, useful thoughts about ourselves: and consequently improve our feelings, our energy levels and our results in the world. To do this, locate the main limiting thought by writing down all the limiting thoughts and noticing the strongest one. Then reverse it. For example, if you locate 'I don't deserve the new promotion' then transform it to 'I deserve my new promotion'. This may feel strange at first but after a very short time it will feel quite comfortable and true for you.

It's a very good idea to focus your energy consciously on the new thoughts: remember you're already always putting enough energy into your thoughts, but now you're being more selective as to which ones you're choosing to determine your feelings, energy levels and results. There is also a wealth of evidence to suggest that our thoughts, beliefs and our self-esteem directly affect our immune system, so feeling better about yourself will actually protect you from illness and disease.

There are two practical ways of doing this. Firstly simply say the new thought to yourself as much as possible, especially immediately on waking and last thing at night. It's very challenging and effective to look into the mirror and speak to yourself in this uplifting way. Then you can actually write to the new thought and write your response to it, as follows:

Affirmation	Response
I deserve my new promotion	Not really
I deserve my new promotion	Maybe

In this way you get to notice and let go of your resistance to feeling good about yourself. Below are listed some uplifting thoughts you will find useful in the area of work, particularly.

- I am good enough at everything I do.
- Because I'm good enough, it's OK for me to make a mistake/ask for support.
- I love what I do and I do what I love.
- My work is my self-expression.
- I express my natural creativity through my work.
- I respect and appreciate myself and so does everyone else.
- I like and approve of myself completely, including in the presence of others.
- I trust myself completely.

2

Setting the scene

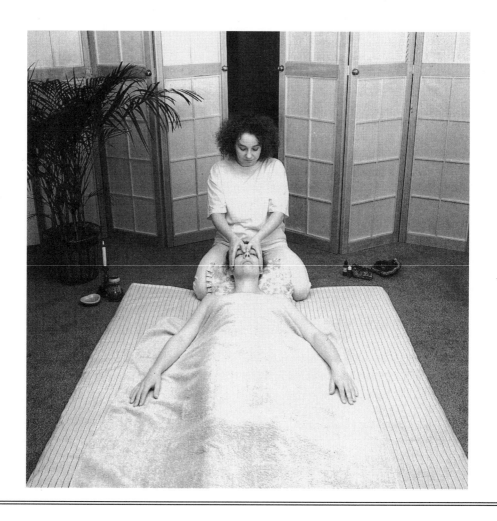

When you are performing massage, it is extremely important to pay attention to the environment in which you will be doing the treatment. There are numerous small details to take into account which will add to the end result. It is highly symbolic to your partner that you have put so much time and effort into creating the nicest possible setting, and it puts the treatment into context.

By spending time in this way, you are conveying to your partner that they deserve to have the best possible room; they are going to be well taken care of and their joy and comfort are a priority for you. The room itself should be immaculate and neatly furnished. The purpose of the treatment is to help clear and clarify the mind: a room which is clear and clutter-free will great assist this. It is perhaps most important to ensure that there will be no intrusions or distractions during the treatment. You will need to take the telephone out of the room and inform children and friends to avoid the room for the treatment time. You will have to take family pets into consideration as it is surprising how animals seek out the quiet atmosphere and tranquillity of the massage room. Choose the quietest room in the house to do the treatment. The next factor to take into account is warmth. Along with quietness, this is the most important consideration. You should heat the room up well before the treatment and make sure that your partner is warm enough throughout. Their body temperature will actually drop during the treatment, so although the room may feel warm enough for you, it may not necessarily be so for them. Keep spare towels and a blanket available. I recommend that you choose some soothing music for the background, as some people may find the silence quite strange and they feel embarrassed and chatter. Having quiet music fills the silence as though there is another person present. However, if your friend is used to receiving massage, they may welcome the deeper silence without music. You may like to enhance the atmosphere by burning essential oils in an oil burner. These are easily available in most health food shops and the aroma of the oils will be appreciated by both yourself and your partner. If you want to use incense, I suggest that you burn it before the treatment rather than during because your friend will be breathing deeply and inhaling incense smoke may prove both irritating and uncomfortable. You will need to ensure that you are wearing suitable clothes. It is essential to be able to breathe and move freely, so wear only loose and comfortable clothes, preferably of a light pastel shade or even white; both of which are uplifting and soothing. You will need to check your fingernails, as it is essential that they are short enough; the shorter the better; you should not wear any hand or arm jewellery. Strong or overpowering perfume should be avoided as this could prove irritating to your partner when they inhale deeply, and if you include essential oils in your oil mixture, you will want the subtle aroma of the oils to dominate the atmosphere. It is also important to consider the lighting in the room. Check whether or not your friend prefers a darkened room. If you are using artificial light, make sure that it is not directly overhead, but discreetly placed. You may even want to use a tinted bulb to add a gentle hue to the room.

The colours in the room will also have an effect. I recommend warm pinks and peaches with towels and sheets of a similar colour. Finally, the finishing touch is to include some plants and a simple arrangement of fresh flowers. These will add a luxurious feel to the occasion. Ideally, your friend should enter the room and feel that their treatment has already begun. They should feel better just by being in the environment itself.

Your attitude

Now that your environment is ideal, you can attend to preparing yourself. The most important part of the preparation is relaxing yourself. The quality and success of your treatment depends to a large extent on how calm and at ease you are. If you have tension in your body and a busy mind, you will more than likely communicate this discomfort to your partner. You want to achieve a state of mind similar to meditation with your thoughts passing by and your focus on your partner and what you are doing. You will want to spend a little time consciously relaxing yourself before you begin a treatment. This can take the form of lying down or sitting comfortably. Take off your shoes and loosen any tight or restrictive clothing. You may like to have melodic music playing very quietly in the background. Take a few comfortable breaths and decide that as you breathe in you are breathing in peace and relaxation. Imagine a 'wave' rippling through your entire body, melting any tension and discomfort. As you breathe out, decide that you are letting go of tension, tightness and anxiety from both mind and body. Allow your thoughts to pass on by; not trying to stop them; not holding on to them; they are like clouds on the horizon, passing you by. Stay in this relaxed mood for a minimum of a few minutes, enjoy how you are feeling and be completely content with it, not feeling you should be any more relaxed than you are. When you feel ready, begin to bring your awareness back to your body; notice the contact of your body on the floor, legs and feet in particular. Wriggle your toes, stretch your legs, wriggle your fingers, stretch your arms and very gently open your eyes. Get up very slowly. This is a very simple relaxation sequence which becomes easier to do and more effective as you practise it. I recommend you take a few minutes to do this before you give a treatment. Done every day for a short time it will bring you noticeable results, such as feeling more relaxed more of the time, and not internalizing turmoil or stress from your environment leaving you better able to cope. Relaxing yourself also encourages you to breathe more thoroughly and deeply. This is particularly important when you are learning to give massage. As with learning any new skill, you may feel a little tense or unsure of yourself and the tendency is to breathe in a very short shallow way, exacerbating any anxiety or tension you may already be feeling. If you begin the treatment relaxed and breathing thoroughly, you are more likely to stay this way throughout. This will benefit both you and your partner. You will finish the treatment feeling relaxed and energized, due to the rhythmic intake of oxygen, and so will your partner. In fact, you will notice that as your partner relaxes, they will automatically breathe more deeply and slowly. You can encourage this practice by breathing audibly during the treatment. This gives your partner permission to breathe deeply and reminds you to as well! If you feel yourself to be a bit nervous during the treatment, it is worth remembering that all caring touch feels good and you can't really make a mistake. It is always quality of touch that makes for a profound treatment. It feels much more satisfying to have 20 minutes of quality touch than an hour's worth of skilfully-performed strokes and routines.

Quality of touch depends on a number of factors: you, the giver, being relaxed yourself, experience and your frame of mind. Relaxation we have already mentioned, and experience comes from lots of practice. The correct frame of mind comes from a clear intention and sense of purpose. This is something you can be in control of and generate right from your first treatment. Be clear on why you are doing the massage and ask yourself what you want to convey to your partner. This will be based on information from them, whether they need to relax, whether they have tension in a particular place. Beyond this, you will also ask the questions 'What do I feel this person needs right now? What do they need to hear or get?' Allow the answer to come before you begin. Perhaps they need reassurance or calmness or to be uplifted. Whatever it is, you need to decide to communicate this quality through your touch to your partner. To do this, you simply close your eyes, visualize this quality as a particular colour that you breathe in and out through your arms and hands to your partner. In this way, you convey a specific quality through your touch and you develop your intuition. Should you find your mind wandering and thinking of other things during the treatment, simply focus your attention back to your partner and communication with them. You should feel relaxed and energized afterwards, as giving the treatment in this relaxed and focused manner is very similar to active meditation. Some people will actually claim to enjoy giving the massage more than receiving it!

Equipment and clothes

The ideal way to give a massage is on the floor on a thick padded futon. Failing this, use some blankets or duvets, but make sure that you and your partner are well protected. I suggest working on the floor for a number of reasons; firstly, it allows you to do a treatment anytime, any place — you are never restricted by not having your table with you; secondly, working on the floor allows you to work with your entire body and to use your body in an effortless controlled way. This means that you can apply deep powerful pressure without getting tired. Just using arms and shoulders, you want to give a dynamic treatment with your whole body; your arms, hands and thumbs being the 'antennae' through which you channel pressure from your whole self. This type of pressure feels very different from a pushing of pressure from the shoulder, which can feel quite invasive and threatening and is likely to provoke resistance from a tense muscle. It is much more effective to persuade tension, gently but firmly to let go and relax, rather than imposing your will on it. This is

a very important aspect of pressure and quality touch. Develop a 'listening' for the body through your pressure. Apply pressure gently and gradually, until you find the point of comfortable depth. Experiment with depth of pressure. You will want to lean into the strokes and apply pressure from your hips. In Oriental philosophy this is the 'Hara' or lower belly area between the navel and pubic bone. This is viewed as the centre of the body's strength and vitality as well as the centre of gravity in the body. Your massage should feel deep and penetrating without being uncomfortable or painful. It is always wise to work with your partner on letting go of holding and tension. It can be that your partner's tension has taken years to materialize in the body and is now an integral part of them and their body. It is therefore more fitting that they let go of it over a period of time and the change is likely to be more permanent. If you suffer from a weak back you may want to buy a massage table; or if your body is stiff you may need to use one until you become more supple and flexible.

Finally, another advantage of working on the floor is that you have a lot more physical contact with your partner. You can kneel alongside them and be in contact with your whole body and not just your hands. This complete contact is an inherent part of the healing process; the more supported your partner feels, the more they will let go. You should avoid chatting during the treatment. This inhibits any deep relaxation on your partner's part and any clear focus on yours. It may be that your friend needs to get something off their chest so be discreet and sense when this is happening. This may be a rare occasion for them to open themselves up and be listened to. Do not enter into conversation but simply listen attentively. At some point you will gently suggest that they bring their awareness to their breath and allow their thoughts to pass on by and breathe in peace and relaxation. Encourage them to breathe deeper by breathing and sighing audibly yourself.

You now need to give your partner some guidelines as to how to get the best out of the treatment. If they are new to massage, they will be completely unsure as to how to behave and how to receive the treatment. Both touch and nudity are classic taboos with many people in the West, so you will have to address 'what to wear' immediately.

Of course it is ideal to have your partner naked so that you can work on all parts without the restriction of clothes. However, your partner may not feel completely relaxed with this, so you always work with and around their preferences. I suggest that you tell them to undress down to what is comfortable, adding that undressing down to underwear is ideal and if they want to undress down to what is comfortable, adding that undressing down to underwear is ideal and if they want to undress completely that is fine also. Check that this actually is fine for you! It is important to take your own feelings and preferences into consideration too. You will find that as people become more comfortable with their body and with you, they will be less reserved about revealing themselves. I feel that it is much better to be understanding in this matter rather than confrontational.

You will also want to explain that you will be checking with them on how your pressure feels; but beyond that they should feel no need to talk but simply to relax. With regard to the release of tension in the body, you may find your partner crying or feeling tearful as you work on a particular area of holding. This is perfectly natural and so simply encourage your partner to relax, and then move on to another part of the body if you are uneasy with this letting go. As your touch becomes more sensitive, you will begin to notice which emotions are held throughout the body. You may even notice that you begin to feel a particular emotion yourself as you work on a certain body part. In this case be careful that you

are breathing fully so as to not hold on to it!

Treatment checklist/guidelines

To sum up:

○ Remember to 'breathe' throughout the treatment.
○ Lean into the strokes; if you feel your shoulders coming into the strokes, relax the shoulders and lean more of your body into the stroke.
○ Keep your movements flowing and rhythmic.
○ Mould your hands around the contours of your partner's body.
○ Move around your partner's body with quietness and respect.
○ Encourage your partner to let you take care of them completely by moving their body with certainty.
○ Keep both hands on the body when massaging.

Use and application of oils

You will use a good quality vegetable or nut oil. I recommend sweet almond, sunflower, safflower or grapeseed. Of these, sweet almond is the richest and grapeseed the lightest. Do not use a mineral oil as this is not only not nourishing to the skin but will actually clog the pores. If you wanted a rich, very nourishing mixture you could also add 20 per cent of one of the following: hazelnut, wheatgerm, apricot, jojoba or evening primrose. The addition of essential oils will enhance the treatment enormously. You need only a few oils to have a variety of aromas and recipes. The most important thing to remember is never to use the oils neat (i.e. not mixed with a vegetable oil), or to take them internally. Although the oils are completely natural, they are also extremely powerful and they do need to be used with respect and care. A whole body treatment will require approximately 25ml of oil to which you will add a total of twelve drops of one or more of the essential oils. A back massage will require approximately 10ml. The guideline is to use one drop of essential oils per 2ml of vegetable oil. Only mix up the amount of oil you want to use for the treatment you are doing. The oils do not keep well once mixed up and the properties evaporate rapidly when exposed to light and air. However, adding 10 per cent wheatgerm oil to your mixture will help preserve it. Keep the mixture in a dark coloured bottle in the fridge. The following oils are probably the most versatile, widely used and easily obtainable. Their specific application will be covered along with other ways to use the oils in later chapters.

Lavender

This is probably the most popular oil. It is good for everything and has the striking ability to enhance the qualities of other oils it is combined with. It calms and relaxes and is wonderful for unwinding and letting go of mental pressure. It is also excellent for insomnia and tension headaches. It is useful for muscle tension where the pain is sharp and piercing. Lavender is most famous for its healing action on burns, in clearing up scars and marks on the skin. It is the exception to the 'never use neat' rule in that it can be safely used by itself. This does not mean that it should be liberally spread over the body, but a few drops applied on the temples for a headache or used locally for a burn is fine. Lavender is probably the oil that you will use more than any other.

Rosemary

This has quite the opposite effect to Lavender in that it is stimulating and more of a 'morning time' oil. As with all the oils its properties work on a mental, physical and emotional level. This means that while it is excellent for stimulating the mind, it is equally useful for sluggishness in the body. In particular it is good for any sinus congestion, fluid retention, cellulite or anything that needs moving. It is valuable for all respiratory problems from catarrh and sinusitus, through to asthma.

Taken as an inhalation, it can often prevent the onset of a cold. Rosemary is the oil to use in a morning time bath or as a 'pick-me-up' after a day's work and before going out for the evening.

Bergamot

This is a glorious 'sunny' oil, refreshing and uplifting and a wonderful antidepressant. It is ideal for any lethargic type of depression as it energizes the whole person. It is also good for infections of the urinary tract, urethritis and cystitis, particularly in treating the root cause of the problem which may lie in anxiety or depression. Bergamot is also ideal for treating acne, oily skin, psoriasis and all infected skin conditions. A word of caution, however. Never use Bergamot before going out in the sun or using a sunbed as it increases the skin's sensitivity to sunlight and can lead to uneven tanning. Bergamot's light citrus aroma makes it ideal for both men and women.

Geranium

This is the all-time balancer. It actually works on a hormonal level to regulate the balance of hormones in the body. It is therefore, of great value in treating premenstrual syndrome and menopause problems. It is also ideal for the type of person who is either very, very up or very, very down but never on an even keel. It is highly likely that Geranium would also prove useful in any case of hyperactivity particularly in children. This balancing property also extends to the skin where Geranium is valuable for skin that is either excessively dry or oily or for dry skin with oily patches.

Camomile

Camomile is a soothing, calming oil which is excellent for both mental and physical irritation or irritated skin, particularly eczema or allergic conditions. Camomile is also valuable for the treatment of internal inflammation, like cystitis, colitis or gastritis. In treating muscle tension or pain, Camomile is best for dull aches and pains. On a mental and emotional level, Camomile is the great comforter to the person who is irritated or nervous.

Neroli

This is the classic stress antidote oil and its subtle aroma is delicate but powerful in its effect. It is particularly useful for nervous highly-strung people who may talk a lot from nervous tension. It is also famous for its importance in skin care. It has the special ability to stimulate the growth of new cells and undoubtedly has rejuvenating effects. It is particularly useful for dry or sensitive skins.

Ylang-ylang

This is a strong-smelling floral oil, quite sweet and concentrated. It is best to use only in small amounts. It has the ability to reduce over-rapid breathing and heartbeat. These symtoms may often arise as a result of anxiety, shock or distress. High blood pressure may also be a feature for which Ylang-ylang is useful.

Rose

This is the ultimate luxurious 'feminine' oil and is also known as the 'Queen of oils'. It is extraordinarily difficult to produce, taking as many as 30 roses to produce one drop of oil. It is therefore extremely concentrated, needing only one drop for an entire body treatment. Rose has a great affinity with the female reproductive system and is used for helping with menstrual difficulties. On the mental and emotional level, Rose is a gentle antidepressant and due to its 'feminine' qualities, is especially useful in treating postnatal depression. It is also excellent for treatment of grief or anger. Rose is also wonderful for skincare, particularly for dry skin or broken veins. Rose is costly, but due to its concentration, will last a long time. It is a very worthwhile investment.

Jasmine

This is known as the 'King of oils' for its qual-ity and its aroma which has a 'masculine' feel in the way that Rose has a 'feminine'. Like Rose, Jasmine is difficult and costly to produce, but lasts a long time due to its concentration. It is also similar to Rose in that it is a valuable uterine tonic, useful for menstrual cramps as well. It is useful when used in childbirth to relieve pain and strengthen contractions. Due to its antidepressant qualities it is useful to relieve postnatal depression. It also helps with impotence and frigidity. It is similar to Bergamot in that it is calming and uplifting, without being sedative. This is most useful in depression which is characterized by lethargy.

Marjoram

Marjoram is a relaxing, warming oil. Its properties are quite similar to Lavender and may be the total ideal alternative for people who prefer a more 'woody' aroma. It is valuable for insomnia and can be combined well with Lavender for this. Due to its warming quality, it is very useful in the treatment of rheumatism, asthma, bronchitis and colds, high blood pressure and heart conditions. It is also well-known for its action on the digestive system. For this reason it is particular useful for stomach tension and menstrual cramps.

In using essential oils it is worth remembering that combined with massage they are spectacular in treating the underlying causes of illness and disease. Use them to relax and uplift, to calm and soothe, to ease tension and anxiety from mind and body. Massage and essential oils are therefore an extremely powerful way to handle the negative effects of stress. In selecting the oils, bear this in mind and do not treat symptoms or serious complaints. You will also notice that the properties of many of the oils overlap so let your partner's preference be your guideline. If they like the aromas and the mixtures, it is more than likely they will benefit from them. If you wish to treat children with oils, you can do so safely as long as you observe a few simple guidelines:

1 Always dilute essential oils before adding them to a bath, using no more than 4 drops in total.

2 Use lower dilutions when preparing a massage oil. Use half the amount of drops that you would normally.

Basic strokes

Touch is instinctive, natural and a skill that we all inherently possess. It may be a skill that we have lost touch with but it is there, however dormant.

There are, nonetheless, systematized routines and applications of touch that have developed through the ages. This system allows us to touch in an efficient therapeutic way. Below is described one such system, the main strokes that make up 'Swedish massage'. All these strokes have specific physiological implications and there is a certain logic to the pattern in which they are performed. Having said this, it is also worth repeating that quality of touch is much more important and effective than technical sophistication. Sometimes, the enthusiastic caring beginner will offer more in their touch than the seasoned veteran who has grown blasé.

Be completely present to your partner and your massage and you really can't go wrong. The strokes will help you gain confidence in your touch as your hands have something specific to aim for. In a short time you will be inventing your own strokes and have quite an extensive repertoire. Firstly you will guide your partner to get comfortable on the futon or surface you are working on. If you are doing an all-over body treatment, you will start on the back, then legs and feet, then your partner will turn over and you will work on neck, head and face, front of shoulders, stomach, arms and hands, legs and feet. Cover your partner with a large towel; most people will prefer to have the areas you're not working on to be covered rather than exposed. This is a generalization, but use it as a safe guideline.

Attunement

Before you begin your treatment, whether it is a complete body treatment or a specific area, always 'attune' to your partner and the treatment you are about to give. This is simply taking a few moments to change gear and move into a mode appropriate to giving a quality treatment. Different types of energy are appropriate to different activities and massage is no exception. Therefore we need to consciously change from one mode to another which facilitates a healing treatment. We need to learn to let go of all previous thoughts and concerns and be completely present to our partner and the treatment. This can be quite a challenge for many of us since we are adept at being concerned with many things at once including past and future. Rarely we do have the opportunity to be solely concerned with the present moment. Assuming that you are giving a back treatment, kneel comfortably alongside your partner's back facing ahead; on his or her left side if you are right-handed, or vice-versa. At this point you can attune with your partner by including him or her in your intention. Speak to your partner in a very soft slow way and follow your own instructions as you speak. It is useful to emphasize some key words and to this end they are written in italics. 'Take a few *comfortable* breaths, allow your body to *sink* into the floor. Let go of everything that has been happening for you. Let your thoughts *gently* pass on by, not trying to stop your thoughts as they come, simply not holding on to them, like clouds on the horizon, passing you by. As you breathe in breathe in *peace* and *relaxation*. Feel that peace and relaxation as a wave *rippling* through your entire body. As you breathe out, *let go* of any tension and any tightness and any anxiety from your mind and your body. Allow it to *pour out of you* as you breathe out.' (You audibly breathe out.)

Make contact

You and your partner are now in a more receptive frame of mind and body to move into massage. The first stroke is simply 'laying on hands'. This first contact is crucial to the tone of the entire treatment and its importance cannot be overestimated. It is the most important stroke of the entire massage. Before you do this you may want to decide what particular quality you wish to convey to your partner through your touch. Simply ask yourself 'What does this person need to hear or accept abut her/himself?' Trust the word or phrase that comes to you and channel this quality through your hands. To assist this, visualize a waterfall of white light, rose pink or golden rays of sunshine above your head pouring in through you. As you breathe in you draw in this healing energy, and as you breathe out, direct it to your centre, rippling through your arms and right into and out of your hands. When you feel ready bring one hand or both to make contact gently on your partner's back while continuing this channel of energy through you to them. Notice their breathing and be open to receive any information from them through this touch. This instinctive diagnosis was something doctors used to do as a preliminary to using a stethoscope. You will want to make contact for a minimum of a minute. You are now ready to apply oil and continue. Roll the towel down to tuck into underwear, making sure the lower back is exposed to be included.

Applying oil

The golden rule here is never ever to apply oil directly to your partner, but always to your palms first with your hands well away from the body. Make sure your hands are warm and rub them together as necessary. Mix enough oil in your palms as is necessary for the particular part that you are about to work on; approximately 3 teaspoonfuls or 10ml is ade-

quate for the back. It is advisable to use a plastic squeezy bottle in the beginning as spillage is reduced to a minimum. It makes a wonderful treat to warm the oil first, especially in cold weather. It is not necessary to maintain constant contact throughout the treatment as long as you move your hands slowly away and back to the body. It may be that your partner will not even notice that you have removed your hands if you do it sensitively. To reduce unnecessary breaks in contact, reapply oil by keeping one hand, palm down, on the body and with the other hand pour the oil on to the back. If all this sounds complicated or time-consuming, don't worry, it isn't! Once you have done it a few times, you will feel completely comfortable and it will make a substantial difference to the treatment. Some people claim that this is the best part of the whole treatment.

Effleurage

This simply means stroking. It is a long gliding stroke performed over the entire area that you intend working on. The purpose of effleurage is to accustom you and your hands to your partner and for your partner to get used to your touch. It allows you to apply the oil to the area you will be working on. Most importantly, effleurage relaxes the muscles so that you can work deeper with following strokes. As you effleurage, your hands will pick up which areas are more taut than others, differences in temperature from one pat of the body to another and provide you with information that will guide the rest of the treatment. Effleurage feels wonderful on the back. Begin kneeling at the side of your partner facing forwards on their left side if you are right-handed, or vice-versa. Tuck the towel into underwear and bring your hands to slowly float down to the lower back (*fig. 1*). Lean in and glide hands up the back around the shoulder and down the sides of the back (*figs. 2 and 3*). You can improvise to a huge extent here and design movements within this basic stroke. The most important aspect is to lean your body into the stroke from your pelvis and to set up a rhythm within the stroke. Close your eyes and immediately your sense of touch will be accentuated and heightened and your partner will notice the difference. Traditionally in the East, blind people were acknowledged as having the most subtle, sensitive and powerful touch. Effleurage will be the most widely used of all the stokes and you will return to it often in between other strokes. This establishes a familiar pattern which can be repeated during the treatment.

Friction

This follows on naturally as your next stroke; as it allows you to work deeper into muscles now you have relaxed the area. Friction is performed with small circular movements with the tips of the fingers, the thumb, or the heel of the hand. This stroke is particularly effective when done along the sides of the spine. Your position should be: inside leg kneeling on the floor alongside your partner's back, facing forwards with the outside foot raised up on the floor. Place hands on either side of the spine, heels of hands almost touching. Lean

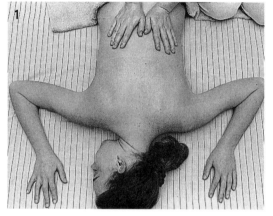

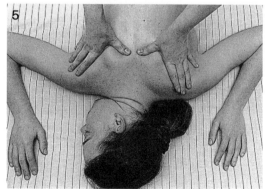

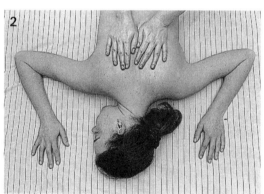

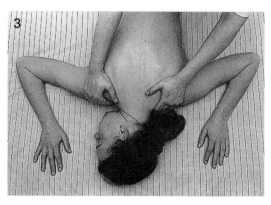

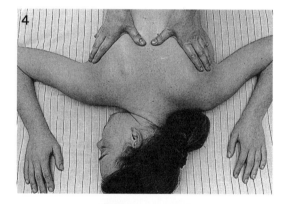

your bodyweight forward into your hands as you spread them across the back: the emphasis is in the heels of the hands. Begin at the lower back, being careful not to apply too much pressure to this sensitive kidney area, and work your way up until you have covered the entire back. You could follow this by leaning your thumbs along the channel either side of the spine (fig. 4). Again your whole hand is in contact but you are leaning pressure specifically into the thumbs. Lean weight into the thumbs and rotate. Begin on the lumbar area and move up to cover the entire back (fig. 5).

Kneading

This stroke is also referred to as petrissage. This is an extremely powerful stroke to get to the very heart of muscular tension and holding. If you perform it correctly, you will be squeezing out tension, toxins, tightness and the very emotional or mental stress behind the discomfort. For these reasons it can feel quite painful and you will have to gauge carefully where the comfortable and useful pain threshold is for your partner. If you get it right they will be letting go, and if you don't, they will be resisting you and holding on tighter than ever. Your touch will be experienced as a threat. Kneading can be applied with great effect to everywhere except the face. It is particularly easy to do on fleshy areas such as the buttocks and thighs. Your position should be: wide knees alongside and facing the area you are working into. Place both hands flat on the skin, fingers pointing towards each other; lean your weight into one hand and push it towards the other while squeezing flesh and muscle between finger and thumb (fig. 6). There should be a gentle swaying to your movement as you lean one side of your body into the stroke and then the other. You may notice a redness appearing beneath your hands and this is a sure indication of the effectiveness of your stroke. The colour is due to blood flowing into the area again once the tense muscle that was blocking it is released. The blood will bring oxygen and nutrients to the area and clear away any stagnation and toxins that have accumulated there.

Pulling

This is another stroke applied over the entire body except for the face. Your position is also as above, wide knees facing the part that you are working on. Place one hand on the far side of the torso or limb, lean your body over and pull up the muscle. Bring your other hand to the same spot to overlap and pull up; repeat this until you have covered the entire side (fig. 7). This can be done as a dynamic vigorous stroke or as a soothing calming one, depending on the speed with which you do it.

Wringing

This is a cross between pulling and knead-

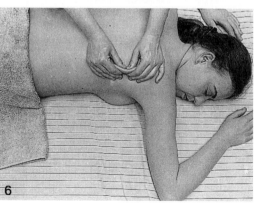

6

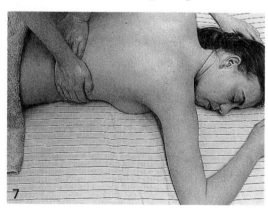

7

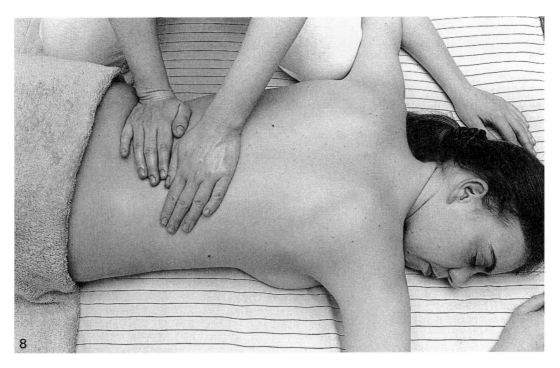

8

ing. The position is again wide knees facing the part to be worked on. The stroke consists of both hands moving simultaneously but in opposite directions. Place hands alongside each other, fingers pointing away from you while you pull back towards you with the other hand (*fig. 8*). Like pulling, this stroke can be either stimulating and invigorating or relaxing and soothing. Either way this is extremely pleasant to receive.

Deep tissue stroke

These strokes are very similar to the friction strokes described earlier, but are for penetrating into deeper layers of muscles and for working around joint spaces. Fingers, thumbs and heels of hands are used. On the back of the leg, for example, kneel by the foot facing towards your partner. Keep the entire hand in contact with the leg; have the emphasis on the heel of the hand. Lean weight gradually into your hands as they glide gradually up the leg (*fig. 9*). This can also be done with

one hand at a time, one hand resting on the ankle. This stroke could equally be applied with thumbs. To do this, the whole hand is again in contact on the leg with the emphasis in the thumbs. Wrap both hands around the calf, thumbs parallel and facing forwards. Lean weight through you as you glide your hands up the leg. To perform this stroke with one thumb, rest one hand on the ankle and place the thumb horizontally across the calf, lean into it and glide up the leg.

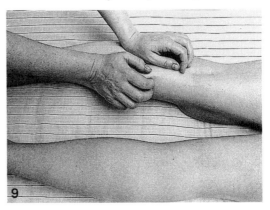

9

Knuckling

This is a wonderful stroke for the upper chest, arms, hands and feet. Curl your hands into loose fists. Place fists, palms facing downwards on the body, rotate the middle sections of the fingers around the area without taking the hands off (*fig. 10*).

Percussion strokes

These are a series of dynamic stimulating strokes. They are ideal for breaking up chronic tension and bringing a lot of circulation and movement into an area that has been tight and congested. This should only be used on padded areas such as thighs and buttocks. Although you can vary the speed with which they are done, the effect will be to invigorate and stimulate. They are not to everyone's liking and would disrupt the silence and flow of a relaxing treatment. Fragile people would not welcome them either. However, it is sometimes appropriate as necessary to wake your friend up at the end of a treatment and this is the sure way to do it! This is particularly relevant if the massage is done in the morning before your friend has to go on to work.

The main essential points to remember with these strokes are that you have a relaxed floppy wrist, have a sense of rhythm in preference to speed, keep your hands close to the body rather than bouncing from a height and keep breathing correctly yourself. It is a good idea to practise these strokes on your own thighs first.

Pummelling

Make your hands into loose fists and bring the sides of the fists down to bounce on to your partner's body. Alternately bounce them up and down (*fig. 11*). Your position for this and all percussion strokes is wide knees facing the thighs and buttocks. Keeping your knees wide allows you to move around the body without feeling imbalanced.

Cupping

Bend your fingers over and bounce gently one hand after the other on your partner's body (*figs. 12 and 13*). The sound you want to produce is that of horses' hooves, going 'clippety clop'. Keep your hands 'cupped' or bent over to avoid slapping your partner, which would feel stinging. Your aim is to create a slight vacuum or air pocket to bring circulation to the skin surface. Cupping can be included on the entire back provided it is done very gently, particularly on the sensitive lumbar region.

Hacking

This is probably the most well-known and notorious stroke of all! It can certainly be the most vigorous and care needs to be taken to apply it successfully. Check that your hands are relaxed and wrists floppy. Bring the sides of your straight hand to bounce down on the body, one hand after the other in rapid succession (*fig. 14*). You will know if your hand

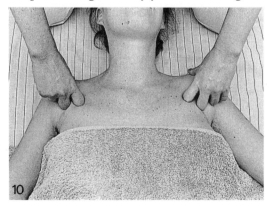

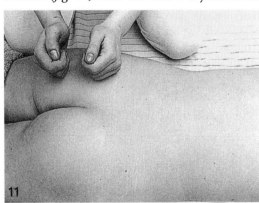

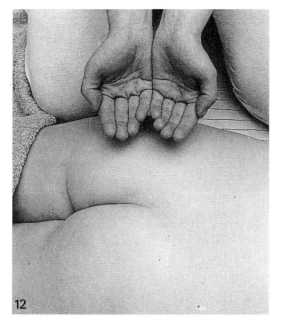

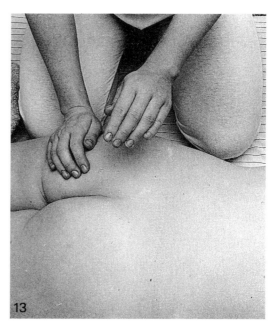

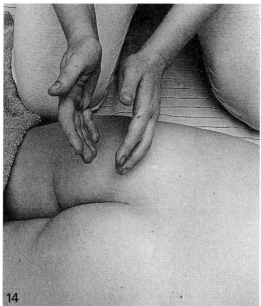

is relaxed if your little finger folds into the hand with each movement rather than remaining erect.

With all percussion strokes, particularly hacking, begin gently and increase your speed gradually. Avoid bouncing directly on the spine.

Completion

To complete your treatment, effleurage over the entire area once again, at least five or six times. Cover your partner up and simply rest your hands on an area you feel drawn to, or move directly to the feet to hold them, and make contact as you did at the outset. As you hold the feet, return to the earlier communication you intended to convey and again breathe this quality in and out through your hands. It is best to remain here to encourage your partner to notice and enjoy how they are feeling. Very gradually bring your hands off the feet. Quietly inform your partner that you are going to wash your hands and reassure them that it is fine to rest for a few minutes. If your partner has fallen asleep, leave them to get up in their own time. It is a good idea to instruct your partner on how to get up from the treatment. Speak the following in a very quiet slow voice, emphasizing the words written in italics: 'Gently bring your awareness to your body, notice the contact of the body on the floor, legs and feet in particular. Wriggle your toes and stretch your legs and feet away from you. Take a few deep breaths. Know that when you get up, you will feel *relaxed* and *mentally alert, relaxed* and *mentally alert*. When you feel ready, roll on to your side and come up *slowly* in your own time. Keep the pleasant feeling you have inside you as you come up.' This instruction is important for a number of reasons. Firstly, your partner may have relaxed very deeply and drifted off into quite another state of consciousness. They need to come back very gradually, just as after deep meditation, otherwise they may experience a stinging headache afterwards. Secondly, you are also giving your partner permission to take a few extra minutes before getting up. Offer your partner a glass of water and take a little time to hear how the massage was for them and to let them know of anything of interest that you noticed: particular areas of tension, how relaxed you felt they were and so on. Finally, a few points you may want to pass on to your friend. Because massage is a luxurious relaxing treatment, its power is often underestimated. If your friend has suppressed tiredness in their body, then they may feel quite tired for a while after the treatment, even for a few days, but after this their energy will be noticeably improved. Massage is also like a dramatic spring clean or fast, which greatly speeds up the elimination of toxins. This may also be the cause of a short bout of tiredness or even a headache. Encourage your partner to allow this process to happen and to avoid taking stimulants such as caffeine or alcohol. Your partner can support this cleaning by drinking no less than a litre a day of spring water. Most of all reassure them that it is fine to feel this tiredness and that it will pass, as many people have a dread of fatigue and not being completely in control. On the other hand, they may immediately experience a tremendous increase in their energy due to the simple fact that it takes a lot of energy to hold a muscle tight. When the muscle relaxes there is then instantly more energy available. Lastly,

it is worth remembering that a tense body may also be a suppressed body. If there are feelings or memories that we are out of touch with, or just underneath the surface, a comforting massage may allow these feelings to come to the surface. As we relax and feel safe, so our bodily defences may melt. If your friend feels tearful or vulnerable after the treatment simply explain what is happening. Encourage them to allow the emotion to keep breathing and let go of it. Sometimes massage provides the spark for people to explore issues which have been previously locked in the body. If this is the case, your friend may well want to have some counselling. With all of the above in mind, it is a good idea to 'time' your treatments a little. For example, if your friend has never relaxed deeply before, is quite hyperactive and drinks quite a lot of alcohol and caffeine, it is advisable to treat them for only thirty minutes to begin with and then gradually increase the duration of the massage as the body and mind get used to the new experience. In time you will get very clear on the likely effects of the treatment on different types of people based on their lifestyle and your heightened intuition. It is a good idea to be in contact with your partner a day after the treatment to look at how they are responding. The healing power of massage is due to its gentle yet profound impact on the whole person.

Basic shiatsu techniques

Most of the preparatory techniques described in the massage section apply to Shiatsu such as preparation of the environment, 'attunement' and making contact. It is usual to include preparatory exercises which focus on loosening and relaxing the body and focusing the attention. These may include simple stretch, breathing and meditation exercises based on Tai Chi, yoga and other systems which combine all these elements. Since Shiatsu works with balancing the body's energy system it is essential for the giver to feel properly 'balanced' themselves before beginning work. The quality of pressure given when one is calm, relaxed and at peace as well as totally alert and purposeful is infinitely more powerful than at any other time. If one feels distracted, scattered, tired or irritable the quality of pressure will suffer accordingly. One's state of mind as well as one's physical state at the time of giving shiatsu will be directly communicated to the receiver through touch. This shows how important it is to be responsible for one's own condition at the time of giving treatment and, by extension, for one's general level of health and well-being. In aiming to relax and revitalize another's mind and body, one must be relaxed and vital oneself.

Shiatsu is visibly quite distinct from Western forms of massage. It involves no actual 'strokes' at all and consists simply of pressure, applied all over the body with the clothes on, to balance the person's energy system by strengthening areas of weakness and releasing areas of tension. This leaves the person feeling relaxed and yet fully revitalized. Traditionally it has been used both for relaxation and for the treatment of many common ailments. It forms an integral part of the Oriental medical system along with acupuncture, moxibustion and herbal medicine and with them, employs clear diagnostic and treatment principles. It has also been used traditionally in the home as a safe and simple 'home remedy'.

Though simple, it has a very varied and dynamic form to it incorporating elements of the ancient massage traditions of Japan (Anma), as well as more modern ones drawn from osteopathic and chiropractic traditions involving stretch and adjustment. The basic principles of pressure are simple and straightforward to apply involving vertical, steady and supporting pressure. Once the pressure has been applied at right angles to the surface of the body it is held for several seconds, penetrating deeply and stimulating the parasym-

pathetic nervous system which calms and relaxes the body. At the same time we must support our body weight over our partner using other parts of our bodies from that which is directly applying the pressure. This may be done by simply using two hands though the knees, elbows and feet are often brought into play as well. The important thing is that two opposite but complementary forces are always applied simultaneously in one movement as you work, the one active (giving) the other passive (sometimes called 'mother'). Mastering the correct use of support and giving pressures is the main challenge facing the shiatsu practitioner. The pressure itself is applied using a variety of different parts of the body as follows:

Thumbs

These are the obvious 'tools' of shiatsu (which literally means 'finger pressure'). They are used for small, precise areas like bone crevices, between muscles and pressure points. These include the head, neck, hands and feet. They are never used alone and full supporting pressure from the fingers and palms is applied along with the thumbs (*fig. 15*). They can become easily tired and it is good to do regular exercises to strengthen them.

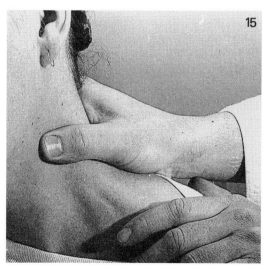

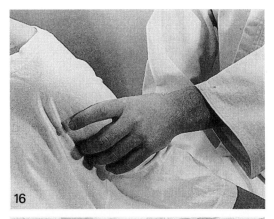

16

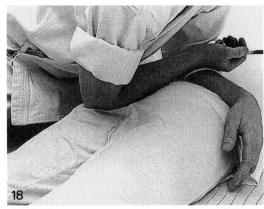

18

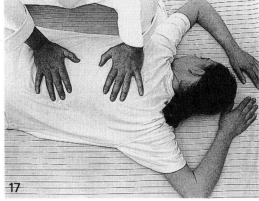

17

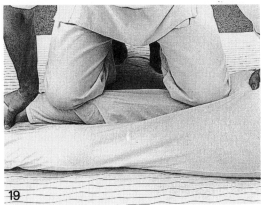

19

Fingers
These are used as explained above for supporting pressure. They are also used for grasping techniques when a whole area is pressed at once such as the arm (*fig. 16*). Otherwise they are principally used for abdominal shiatsu and diagnosis.

Palms
Probably the most widely used technique in shiatsu. Very relaxing and sedating. Strong pressure can be used but well spread out over the whole hand. The palm should mould itself to the contours of the area being worked on though more often this technique is used on fairly flat areas such as the back (*fig. 17*). The heel of the palm can be used more precisely though the fingers always remain in close contact with the surface being worked

on. Palming pressure can be used to 'prepare' an area to be worked on as well as go over an area which has just been worked on, rather like effleurage in massage (see page 28).

Elbows
More properly it is actually the forearm which is used, only occasionally is the point of the elbow itself used since it gives very strong, focused pressure. Mainly used for large, muscular areas such as the back, legs and buttocks where pressure can be fairly deep and strong. It is straightforward leaning pressure, using the other hand/elbow for support (*fig. 18*).

Knees
Despite their size the knees can give very soft, relaxing pressure, partly because it is spread over a large area. However the supporting

pressure (from the two hands) must be very firm and stable so the movement can be slow and controlled (*fig. 19*). Care must be taken in applying the pressure since the knees are less sensitive and therefore it is less easy to gauge the correct amount of pressure to give. They are mainly used on large, soft areas like the hips and legs and sometimes the arms.

Feet

The feet are highly sensitive areas of our body. They carry our entire weight around most of the time and form our direct link with the ground beneath. It is natural that they should be used in shiatsu to give pressure. In many other massage forms they are used extensively especially in Indian massage some of which is done entirely with the feet. Almost any part of the body can be pressed by the feet though it is a technique requiring good balance and coordination. One simple technique which is very effective is 'walking on the feet.' Simply apply pressure with one or both feet to the upturned soles of your partner's feet (*fig. 20*).

A combination of any or all of the above techniques may be used in a shiatsu treatment. They may be applied in any of the 4 main positions, lying on your side, front or back and sitting up. One principle that is common to them all however is the use of relaxed body weight. This always involves having a good, firm base with steady knee and feet positioning, moving from the hips or 'hara' region (the energy centre in the lower abdomen) and applying the three basic principles mentioned: vertical, steady and supporting pressure. Beyond this, there is little other 'technique' involved in shiatsu and it is as important to have a 'beginner's mind' and pure intention as a variety of professional techniques. Often simple, honest shiatsu is the most effective.

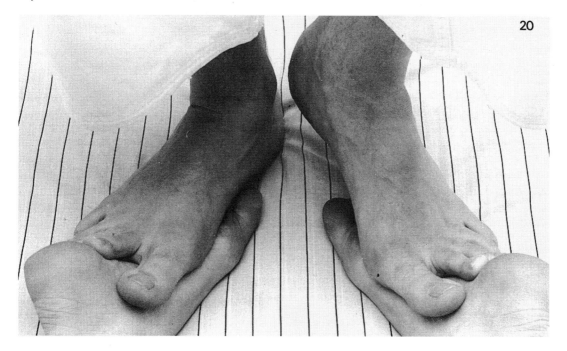

20

3

At work

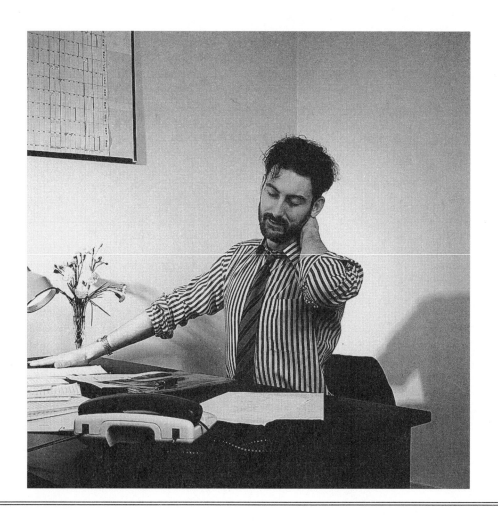

It is natural for humans to work. For as long as they have been on the earth, humans have sought to play an active role in creation. Whether as a direct response to external stimuli or as a conscious creative act, our evolution has depended on our effectiveness and inventiveness at work. But the word has gained unfortunate connotations, in that it implies disagreeable effort and exertion.

Work, in fact, has become a dirty word, associated with an unpleasant reality in life. Tolerated at best, but more often despised and resented. A recent survey in the United Kingdom reported that 90 per cent of people are unhappy with their jobs. Our language reflects this negative appreciation of work and its role in society. We use terms like 'labour intensive', 'hard labour', and 'workaholic'. Compare this with the terminology we have for play: gentleman of leisure, time off [work], holiday (from Holy Day — the seventh day when God rested after creating the earth).

Even the word recreation suggests that somehow we need time off work to be fully creative. This has certainly not always been the case. The first organized work that people probably undertook once they moved from a nomadic lifestyle was agriculture, and as any farmer today will tell you this work is indeed a 'labour of love'. In this context work performed many functions, not simply the bread-winning one. It was an efficient form of physical exercise, a means of bringing people together for a common purpose (the harvest), as well as the appreciation of nature and the environment. Then humans had all the benefits of a harmonious lifestyle — regular hours, healthy meals, exercise, communion with nature.

In modern society, work seems to be synonymous with survival. We seem to be back to a caveman attitude of working just enough to stay alive. This poor image of the value of work within our society can be understood in terms of the huge environmental, social and economic changes brought about by industrialization and the move toward the cities. Our work space has been drastically reduced. We have been taken out of our natural surroundings and placed in artificially lit, poorly-ventilated and cramped surroundings. We work shifts and at any hour of the day or night. Our work environment is often polluted and there is little or no opportunity to exercise. Worse still, many feel that their work is insignificant or they cannot see that they are making any contribution. They see themselves merely as another cog in the machinery which will continue with or without them. Perhaps this fact alone — the inability to make a difference in their immediate environment — is responsible for the poor way in which we seem to regard work.

Work which is desperately repetitive, or which requires no skill, where movement may be restricted; where there may be high levels of noise or bright lights, where there may be a high level of risk, or simply where one feels out of touch; where the level of social interaction is so poor that one is lonely, isolated and bored: these are all possible factors contributing to the poor image of work in our society. Link these factors with the increasing levels of competition for work and within work itself, to the pressures on men and women to succeed, to the lure of status and power with which we too readily equate work, and all the basic ingredients of stress and its often disastrous effects on health are firmly in place.

The effects of stress in the workplace are well documented. Stress can cause the straightforward symptoms of the 'emergency response', general strain and tension or more severe problems such as high blood pressure, hypertension, migraines, eating disorders including anorexia, palpitations, anxiety attacks, insomnia, depression, ulcers and many more. The links between stress and cardiovascular disease are especially well-documented. Long-term effects of stress on the immune system are certain to be proved devastating.

It is worth noting the mechanics of stress here since a thorough understanding of our body's reaction to stressful stimuli often increases our awareness and ability to cope with the situation. Dr Hans Selye was the first to carry out systematic research on stress and its effects on the body, defining it as a person's inability to adapt naturally to a given situation. This process may vary tremendously from one person to another, which is why stress itself is such an intensely personal phenomenon. Naturally, food or sleep deprivation or intense pain may be stressful in themselves but even pain is experienced differently by each of us according to our thresholds. In short, very few phenomena or situations could be described as being stressful in themselves. Instead, we must examine our ability to deal with changes in our circumstances and adjust to them appropriately. The extent to which we are able to do this successfully may determine the levels of stress we experience. For example, some people who move jobs every two or three years apparently cope with the upheaval of changing home, friends, schools and environment. For others, even the thought of moving away from the house they have lived in all their lives would cause considerable stress and even illness. Some women clearly suffer terrible stress during menstruation while others apparently experience none.

It is impossible to define which situations actually cause stress. It is nevertheless becoming very clear to us that there are obvious, definable feelings and signs of being under stress. The things to watch for are any sudden changes in behaviour or emotion. You may do things you never used to do or stop doing things you enjoyed before. You may become erratic, irritable, edgy or unpredictable in your behaviour. You may feel relationships difficult and your libido may decrease. You may experience feelings of tension and 'uptightness', finding it difficult to relax. Physically, your eating and sleeping habits may become erratic, you may get dizzy or feel nauseous, even frightened or panicky. Generally you may feel driven or under pressure and this will often end in frustration and anger.

These are all signs of the so called 'stress response'. When we feel under stress our body responds by releasing adrenal hormones which essentially prepare us for 'fight or flight'. This is a natural function which affords all animals protection against danger and enhances metabolism to allow for defence or escape. This could be called 'healthy' tension, a measure of which is needed for proper performance of the organism. Prolonged stress, however, causes continued release of corticosteroids, the so-called 'stress hormones' of the body, which can suppress the immune system causing reduced resistance to disease. It is possible that immune deficient diseases such as ME and AIDS could be better understood in this light.

Physical and psychological stress are always characterized by an increased heart rate, blood pressure, breathing rate, hypertension, muscle tension, sweating, state of mental arousal and adrenalin flow. All of these, if prolonged, can cause heart and kidney disease, stomach ulcers, ulcerative colitis, menstrual disorders and sterility. Links between stress and mature-onset diabetes have been suggested. The obvious connection between stress and mental and emotional disorders is well known, including addictive behavioural problems, such as alcoholism, drug dependence, anorexia and bulimia for example.

Allergic conditions such as asthma have been linked with stress as have arthritis and even cancer, both of which have been described as 'angry' diseases — anger being a very common response to stress. Clearly we must not attribute all disease purely to stress. Diet, exercise and environmental factors obviously play a huge role. But it is safe to say that stress contributes to a large number of diseases, particularly modern degenerative ones such as heart disease, which is still the biggest single killer in Western countries today. On a more general, day-to-day basis, stress probably has affected all of us at one time or another and we may have experienced it as tiredness, lack of energy and general irritability. Many of us have come to accept and put up with this daily reduction in our performance at work and at home and the resulting decrease in the quality of our lives. And yet, with some simple alterations to our diet, to how we exercise and rest or relax and, perhaps most importantly, to how we see and feel about ourselves and our work, we could easily enhance the overall quality of our lives.

Perhaps the most significant statistic to emerge from the wealth of research into stress and its effect in the workplace is the fact that stress levels are strongly affected not only by the kind of work people do, but by the degree of control they have in that work. People with a very low level of control in their work are subject to extremely high levels of stress with the accompanying risks to their health. In other words, people are stressed by the inability to assume responsibility and make decisions about the work they do. This again points to our basic desire firstly to create or contribute something through our work and secondly to be acknowledged for it. Work is not therefore merely a form of earning our daily bread. It provides a far more significant social function — one of providing a means of basic communication, of physical and mental exercise, of fun, accomplishment and contribution to ourselves, our families and our environment.

We are clearly out of touch with this role of work within our lives. The ways in which we might gain access to it again are many and varied. First and foremost, we must learn to love our work.

A major part of our life centres around work: our careers, our workplace, our ambitions. To a large extent our life is shaped by the work we do: our income dictates the area we live in our home and our leisure time. Much of our life is determined by this one area called work.

Self worth

In the present climate, the work we do has also come to define who we are as individuals. When we are introduced to someone the obvious question is always 'and what do you do?' 'What do you do?' has become who we are. Being 'successful' has become synonymous with the job and how highly rewarded we are. So it is no wonder that in our Western culture we as individuals often judge our 'success' or 'failure' as human beings in direct relation to work. For men in particular, being successful also extends to providing a comfortable material base for their family. Even though many women also work, our culture still holds the male responsible as the breadwinner in a two-parent household. Women are now in a double bind situation. They are now facing the same challenges and rewards as men but at the same time are still held responsible or hold themselves responsible for the well-being of home and family. Indeed, in some industries it is clear that women do not merely have to be equal to men for the job but actually much superior, due to longstanding prejudice in these areas.

Work is no longer a simple activity we do to earn money, but something that shapes how we see and value ourselves and to a large extent how others see us. Our self-worth and self-esteem can often rely on recognition and promotion at work. Healthy competition can easily turn into constant anxiety where we are never sure we are good enough and caught up in trying to prove that we are. We need to find a balance where we can enjoy work as a challenge and opportunity, which supports and sustains us in many ways, but which does not determine our total worth as a human being.

Exercise and work

It is important to balance intense and static working conditions with a good measure of active exercise. Whilst this may be done in the early morning, after work or at weekends at clubs or gyms, as well as at home, it is important to integrate some exercise into the working day. Even a few minutes every hour or after lunch is enough to relax and revitalize yourself ready for resuming work with renewed vigour. Our concentration span is enhanced by regular breaks and by gentle stretch and relaxation exercises.

Any exercise undertaken must not be rushed or overdone as its purpose will be undermined. Since, as we have seen, many of the problems we experience in the workplace are a direct result of stress-related conditions, we may reasonably concentrate our recommended exercises on reducing such stress-related symptoms as have been mentioned. Probably the most general ill-effects of stress that can effectively be combated by regular exercise are heart disease and low energy and vitality.

Specific exercises at work

During set breaks or at regular intervals during the day, make time for some of the following simple exercises. They concentrate mainly on the neck, shoulders, face and head, since poor posture at work often leads to stiffness and tension in those areas.

Exercises (see chapter 10)
1) Shoulder lift and drop (see page 160). 2) Shoulder rotation (see page 159). 3) Neck stretches (see page 160). 4) Arm over the back of head and side stretch (see page 158). 5) Arm across chest closed and open (see page 157). Twist body. 6) Eye movements (see page 161). 7) Lip and mouth movements.

Self-massage
1) Palm massage squeezing tops of shoulders concentrating on GB 21 with fingers (*figs. 21 and 22*). One hand at a time.

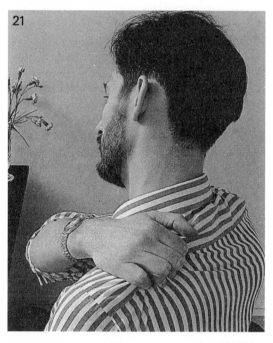

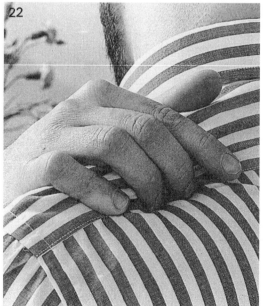

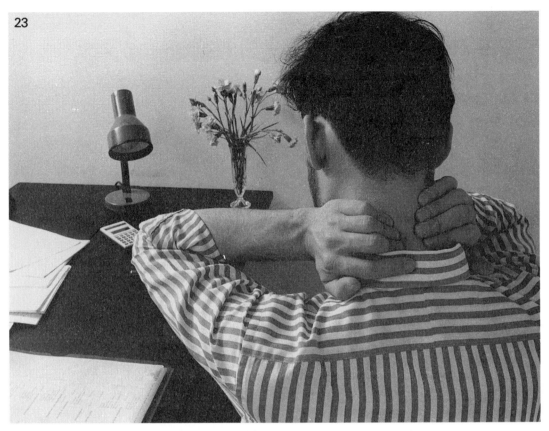

2) Finger massage of back of neck. Double handed (*fig. 23*).

3) Thumb pressure under back of skull concentrating on GB 20 (*figs 24 and 25*).

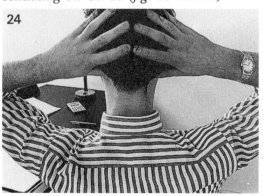 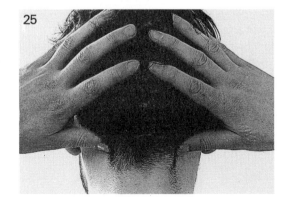

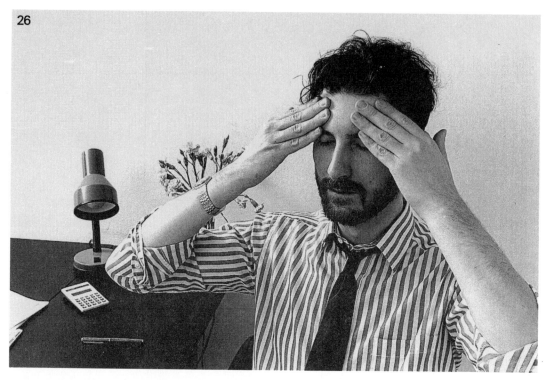

4) Finger massage all over face and forehead and ears (*figs. 26, 27 and 28*).

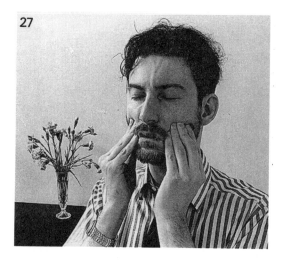

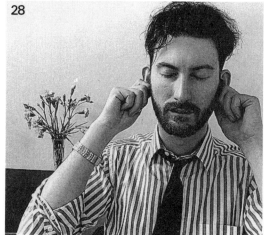

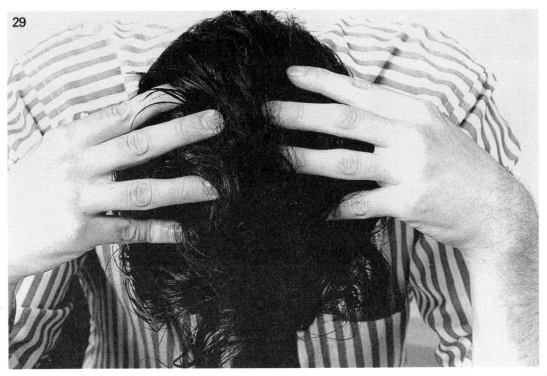

5) Rubbing of scalp (*fig. 29*).

6) Percussion of neck, shoulders, etc (*fig. 30*).

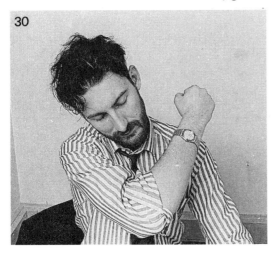

Meditation

Take shoes off. Loosen any constricting clothes, particularly around the waist. Close your eyes. Notice how you're feeling. Sit comfortably with hands in lap or on knees. If you share an office you'll need to tell them you're taking a few minutes' 'shut-eye'. Put a notice on your door if your have your own office and make sure the telephones are being handled for you. Bring your awareness to your breath. Notice the contact of body on your chair and your feet on the floor. Take a few comfortable breaths. Imagine you're breathing in feelings of peace and well-being and as you breathe out let go of any tension, tightness, or anxiety from your mind and body. Allow that discomfort to pour out of your body (*fig. 31*).

Notice the rise and fall of your breath. If there is anywhere in your body that still feels tense or uncomfortable, bring your awareness to that part and bring those feelings of well-being and peace to that part. Allow that ten-

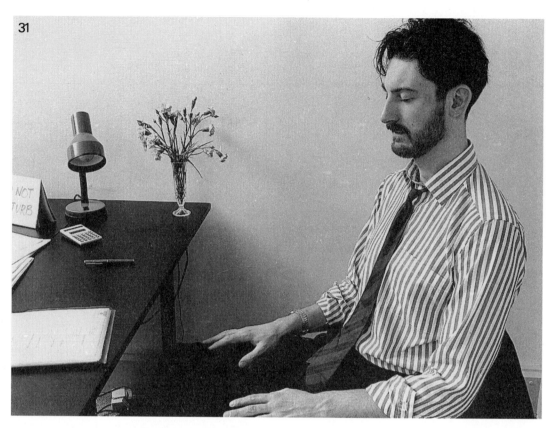

sion to pour out as you breathe out. Give yourself permission to make a 'sighing' sound as you do this. Take the next few minutes to recognize and enjoy how you're feeling with your awareness on the gentle rhythm and flow of your breathing. When you're ready bring your awareness back to your body. Notice again the contact of your body on the chair and feet on the floor. Wriggle your toes and stretch your legs and feet away from you. Wriggle your fingers and stretch your arms and hands up and away from you. Give yourself a really good stretch! Gently open your eyes. This exercise need only take five minutes, but may prevent an energy 'slump' and revitalize you for the rest of the day.

Massage and Shiatsu at work

The self-massage techniques described above are perfectly effective in themselves but there can be no substitute for the quality of another person's touch. We recommend that you experiment at work with the practice of massaging your friends and colleagues. Just a short, simple neck and shoulder rub can produce excellent results, relaxing and invigorating your partner and improving their powers of concentration.

This is quite a common practice in Japan where company employees are famed for their morning exercise routines and where massage for 'Kata Kori' (or stiff shoulders, a recognized medical condition in Japanese society) is often practised in the office. You don't have to be experienced at this most natural of actions and the following are some simple sequences to follow. Remember to refer to Chapter 2 for the basic strokes if you need to.

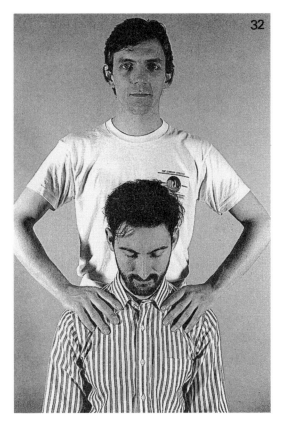

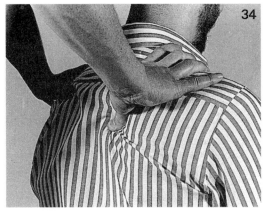

3. Support the back with one hand and lean the thumb of the other into one side of the upper back, in between the spine and shoulder blade. Work over this area thoroughly, leaning thumb in and rotating in a small circle. Repeat this over the entire area. Change support hand and repeat on other side (fig. 34).

Sitting position
1. Make contact on the shoulders (fig. 32).

2. Gently at first, and then more firmly, squeeze the shoulder muscles (fig. 33).

4. Rest one hand on one shoulder and vigorously rotate the heel of the other hand on upper back (fig. 35).

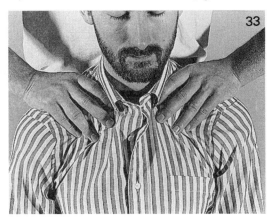

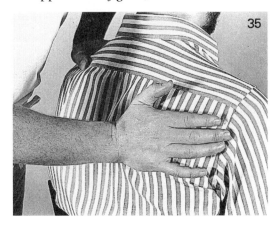

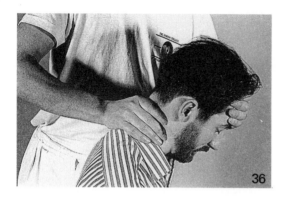

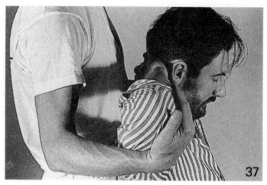

5. Stand to the side of partner. Let the forehead drop into one hand and lean the other hand into the neck, squeezing the muscles between thumb and fingers (fig. 36).

6. Ask your partner to clasp their hands behind their head. Clasp your hands around the elbows and on your partner's out breath, slowly bring the arms back into a comfortable stretch. Repeat and bring arms to rest on their lap (fig. 37).

7. Sweep your hands slowly over your partner's forehead, head, neck and upper back. Repeat 5 times and finish by squeezing the arms (figs. 38, 39 and 40).

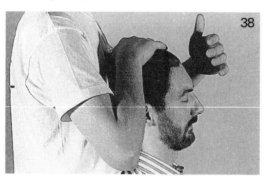

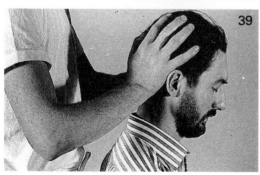

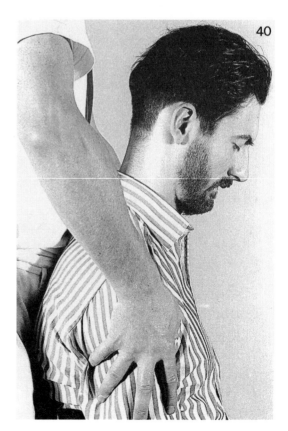

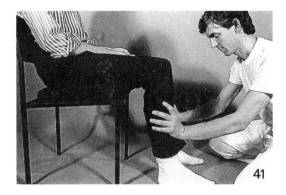

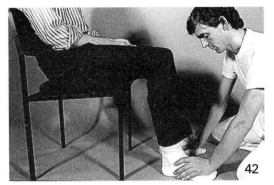

8. Brush down legs and hold feet for a few moments (*figs. 41 and 42*).

Points
Giving Shiatsu in the sitting position is an excellent way to do work on your partner's head, neck and shoulders. Use the simple sequence described above to relax your part-ner first and then use the following points which are usually tight on most people:

Neck Meridians most usually affected in this area are: Gall Bladder, Triple Heater, Small Intestine and Large Intestine. Concentrate on: GB 20 (*fig. 43*), SI 16 (*fig. 44*), SI 17 (*fig. 45*), LI 17 (*fig. 46*), LI 18 (*fig. 47*), TH 16 (*fig. 48*), UB 10 (*fig. 49*).

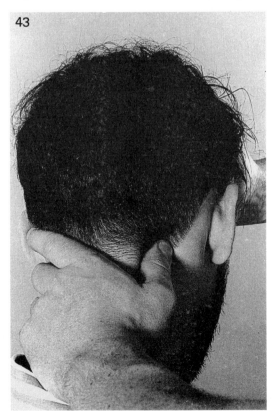

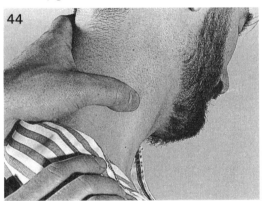

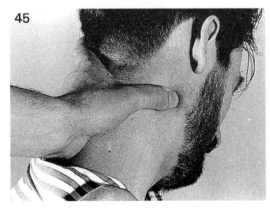

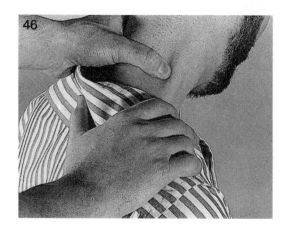

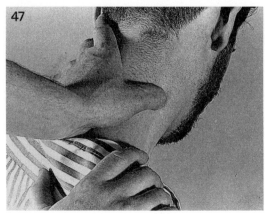

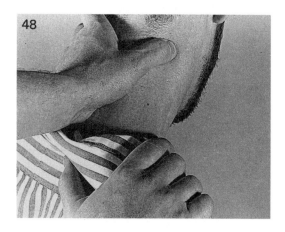

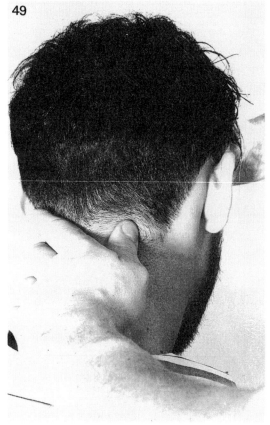

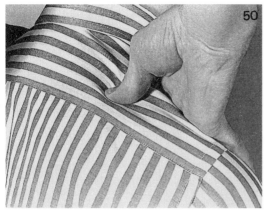

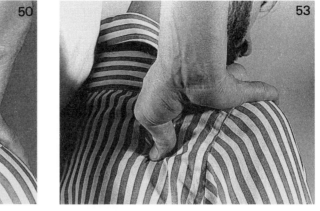

Shoulders Concentrate on points along the same meridians: GB 21 (*fig. 50*), SI 9 (*fig. 51*), SI 10 (*fig. 52*), SI 11, (*fig. 53*), SI 12 (*fig. 54*), SI 13 (*fig. 55*), SI 14 (*fig. 56*), LI 16 (*fig. 57*), TH 15 (*fig. 58*).

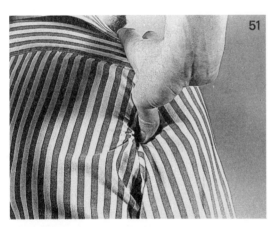

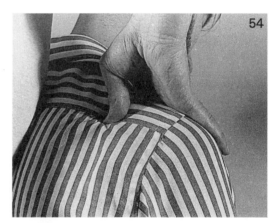

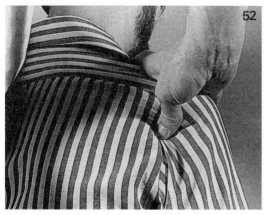

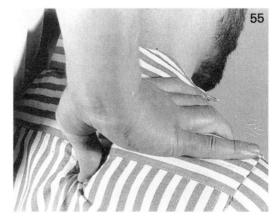

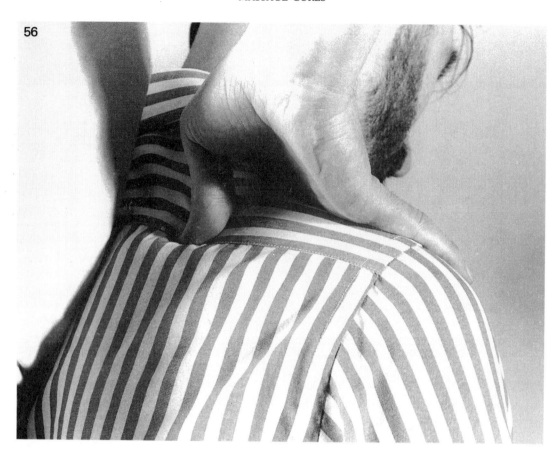

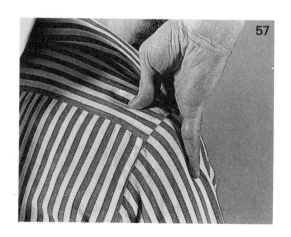

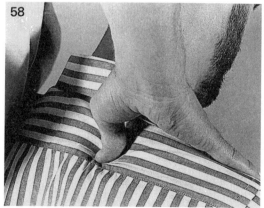

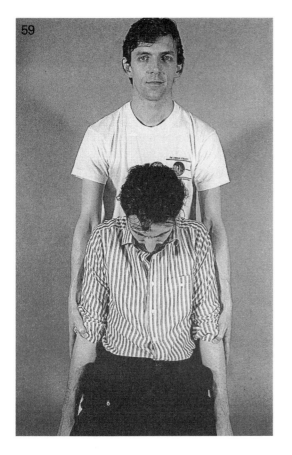

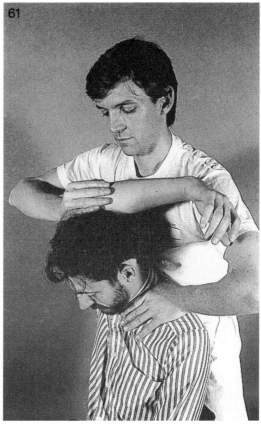

Arm rotation and stretches will also loosen the shoulders considerably (see above under work exercises, some of which can be done by a partner — *figs. 59, 60 and 61*).

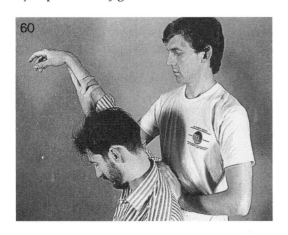

Self-esteem

It is common to see work as something you have to do but which you don't actually enjoy, so you may find yourself wishing the time away, daydreaming and feeling terrible on Mondays and only looking forward to Fridays. In fact there is the saying 'Never buy a Monday or Friday car'! This would suggest that our attention on these days is anywhere but at work. This is extremely sad as we spend a large part of our life at work and therefore not enjoying ourselves. It also means we are not making the contribution in our work that we might do. We have the power to alter radically how we perceive and experience ourselves and our work. Perhaps we could make an experiment called 'Finding fulfilment at work' where we take total responsibility for inventing and sustaining excitement and fulfilment at work. The person who stands to gain the most from this experiment is yourself. Your behaviour will have a 'rippling' effect on everyone around you and on your organization/company as a whole. But above all, you will enjoy increased aliveness and optimism. Your enthusiasm will also create unforeseen opportunities for you and new possibilities and promotion where before you felt buried and resentful. Some supportive thoughts that will propel your actions are:

○ I am ready to let go of my resentment towards my work/boss/employees.
○ I love what I do and that love is opening up exciting opportunities.
○ I always have enough time to do everything I want to do.

It's also very important to be in touch with a major goal which moves you in a certain direction. If, for example you would ultimately like to be a company manager, partner or director and you are currently working as the secretary/toilet cleaner, see yourself as being in training for your projected job. Work at a plan that has you moving from one area to the next, gaining mastery and valuable experience with each move. You also need to check that your work and your goals are really your own and not those of your parents or your teachers. Be honest with yourself and admit what you really want to do.

Even if your decision may incur intial disapproval, you will make a major contribution through doing it rather than doing what was expected of you. However, we can still make the best out of the present work we are engaged in. It is important to appreciate and do our best at our current work as that is our training at that present moment; there is no advantage in negating its value. We can always find things to value and learn about and be grateful for in whatever we do. This is an attitude that can be cultivated and that brings great rewards. It is the direct opposite of resentment — of feeling sorry for ourselves as victim. The outlook and attitudes we choose to nurture and project actually reap their harvest: if we project appreciation and gratitude we will have more in our life to appreciate and be grateful for. It is exactly the same for resentment and bitterness.

We could benefit enormously from seeing work as an opportunity for our self-expression. We are all endowed with certain gifts and talents. We need to acknowledge and appreciate these talents and find or invent a means of channelling or diverting these qualities.

It is when we are aligned with our particular desires and abilities that we have most to offer our fellow human beings. We could call contributing to others and our environment by the name 'work'. In this way we get to be able to experience ourselves making a difference to our world and enjoying our life fully at the same time. Self-expression, fun and financial reward become indistinguishable and inseparable.

1) Do what you're good at and enjoy.

2) Do it well — to the best of your ability or not at all.

If you are not happy in your work, do something about it. Find another job. For it is not just you who will be miserable but everyone around you. We have all the experience of being at the mercy of a resentful, disgruntled waitress who has spoilt a meal and occasion for us. That person might be completely different if she were doing something else that she really wanted to do.

It is very easy to find excuses why things are not possible, but if our happiness and life are at stake, then surely we will find a way to overcome any obstacles to create opportunities. We all know someone who has succeeded in the most adverse conditions.

Money — quality of life

Work and money are inseparable. Because of this we often see work as something we do solely for money, and choice plays no part in the matter. It may be that we could never envisage being paid for enjoying ourselves, or that we'd feel uncomfortable at receiving money for something we'd regard as a hobby. We need to let go of this way of thinking because it will prevent us finding satisfaction and joy when we receive payment. Conversely we may need to examine how attached we are to a particular sum of money if we prevent ourselves doing something we really want to do that might pay less. This is clearly a question of quality of life.

We increasingly hear stories of courageous individuals who give up lucrative but deadening work to fulfil their dreams in jobs that pay much less. These people would say their life is much richer than ever before.

These affirmations will support you in doing work that you love to do.

○ It's OK for me to be paid for enjoying myself.
○ People love to pay me large sums of money for my loving work.
○ I love what I do and that love brings me an abundance of money.

When we enjoy what we are doing we are much more likely to receive more money than before. This is clear to see if we are self-employed. We do a better job and people appreciate the service we provide. People who are good at their work usually love what they do.

Essential oils

Depression/tiredness Bergamot, Rose, Basil, Rosemary, Lavender. Any of these oils can be used in massage, baths or hanky inhalations.

Monday-morning feeling Bergamot, Rosemary. A morning bath in one or both of these will brighten up the day for you.

Impatience/irritability Camomile, Rose, Lavender, Neroli. All of these oils are soothing and calming. Bath, hanky inhalation.

Insomnia/worry Camomile, Lavender, Marjoram, Bergamot. Bath, hanky inhalation.

Muscular tension Marjoram, Lavender. Bath, compresses.

All the above conditions can be greatly relieved by the oils being applied through massage, either self-administered or preferably by a caring therapist.

Bach flower remedies

○ **Lack of confidence:**	Larch
○ **Worry/insomnia:**	White chestnut
○ **Fear of the future/ pessimistic:**	Aspen
○ **Uncertainty regarding one's path in life:**	Wild oat
○ **Monday morning feeling:**	Hornbeam
○ **Overwhelmed:**	Elm
○ **Resentment/feeling powerless:**	Willow
○ **Exhaustion:**	Olive
○ **Impatience/irritability:**	Impatiens

One remedy, or a combination of no more than three of the above, can be taken.

4

Couples

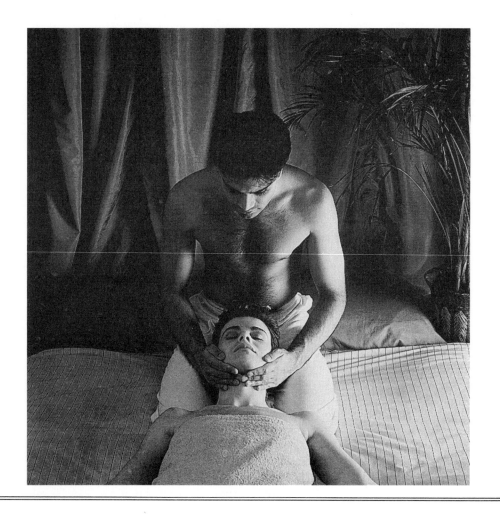

Touch and massage have traditionally played a prominent role in all human relationships, especially intimate ones. Couples have used massage in the art of love-making for thousands of years and this is well documented in Taoist sexual practices (from ancient China), in the Hindu *Kama Sutra* as well as in modern, post-Freudian literature. The application of aromatic oils and elixirs have traditionally been seen as accepted acts of foreplay.

Since the late 1960s we have undergone a sexual explosion where all our social rules and codes have been challenged and many traditional habits have changed beyond recognition. These changes have created enormous freedom for both men and women: women no longer face the same double-standard prejudices as they used to. There is a lot more freedom too for homosexual relationships to be accepted into society. These extraordinary changes will require radical readjustments in our society.

These days however, in an increasingly desensitized, non-tactile world, we have literally lost touch with this acceptable form of of sensual touching. Sex is often reduced to a mechanical, crude device for gratifying our increasingly complex psychological and physical needs. The full meaning and value of intercourse, of which the sexual act is only a part, has been devalued. In part this is due to our changing attitudes about touch in general. The physical act of touching another human being is often laden with perceived rather than intended sexual innuendo. Taboos have grown up around our inadequacies and embarrassment about touch as well as our preconceptions. Homosexuality, age differences, colour, race, religion — all have associated touch taboos based on our equating touch with sexual relationships.

Natural, spontaneous touch has therefore very limited opportunity to express itself and thus we find that within socially acceptable relationships it is often exaggerated and over-

indulged. Young teenage couples are often overtly tactile: kissing and cuddling in public. In some cultures this public touching is commonplace, since it is not tolerated in the home. In Russia and China, for example, the parks are full of kissing couples. In Western cultures, touch has become synonymous with sex and young couples rarely take the time to develop any real level of relationship before they have sex. Sex has become an end in itself, almost the factor which defines the relationship rather than an expression of it. Openness around sex has brought with it pressure for individuals to include sex in their relationship: otherwise we believe there is something missing. There is rarely any old-fashioned courting where boy and girl get to know each other over a period of time: then, sex had a role to play in that it gave physical expression to a relationship that had already been nurtured and built. All too often sex becomes confused with impressing one's partner and has very little to do with a shared loving experience. Indeed it may be that what we call freedom has become another form of pressure for many people, and with it has come a new set of rules. Both men and women may feel at odds with the social codes if they do not comply with having sex early in their relationship, or with a number of different partners. Men, in particular, experience a lot of peer pressure to conform to the role of constantly expressing their virility. Women are bombarded with images of how the ideal woman should look and this puts enormous pressure on their relationships.

The increase in the incidence of AIDS is altering our sexual outlook once again. We are seeing a decrease in the allure of promiscuity and numerous partners: long-term relationships and commitment are fast becoming fashionable again. This unprecedented transformation of our social and sexual roles has brought difficulties, uncertainties and insecurities. All change, whether good or bad, is by its very nature challenging and requires healthy adaptation. The present time is something of a testing period and we are all the guinea pigs in this extraordinary experiment. There are no blueprints or maps for us to follow. We are truly in charge of inventing our relationships. We have an opportunity to design our lives in a way that we can be totally responsible for.

The last 30 years have heralded some phenomenal changes in our culture. This is to be most clearly found in the radical transformation of the roles of men and women. Gone are the familiar, clearly-defined roles of homemaker; wife and mother; and the man as breadwinner, husband and father. Since the late 1950s women have challenged their traditional but confining roles and have made astounding advances into the traditionally male workplace and public life in general. Being 'a housewife' is no longer an occupation as it once was. Labour-saving devices and convenience foods have rendered much housework obsolete.

Woman are now faced with the task of competing with men in the workplace and handling the responsibility of home and children as well. For many women, their life has become a complex juggling of demands and tasks, each apparently equally essential. This hectic schedule creates enormous stress and puts untold pressure on a relationship. A busy career-woman who is also a mother and chief housekeeper may have little time or energy left at the end of a busy day for either herself or her partner.

Men too, have a huge adjustment to make in how they think of themselves and their role in relationships. Their importance and contribution is now largely shared by their partner, and they are no longer the sole or main provider for the family. Nor indeed can they expect to have their needs met as their own fathers did. Men cannot expect regular meals on the table or their domestic needs rigorously taken care of. They may be expected to participate in the day-to-day running of the household and play a more active role in the bringing up of their own chidren. Men can no longer see themselves as the paternalistic figures they once were for women. As women have achieved financial independence, so men's relationship to women has fundamentally altered. Women are no longer bound to men for their material well-being.

The changing roles of men and women are partly responsible for some of the attitudes towards relationships. Women's liberation, almost an antiquated expression in itself, has called for much readjustment in conventional relationships. Added stress has been placed on both partners since women became more career-oriented. For the woman, the risk of discrimination at work and the possible double pressures of career and domestic work combine to affect seriously her attitudes towards men in general, and thus her partner. One result is often reduced libido. Similarly, the men may feel threatened by the idea of equality in the partnership and this may cause feelings of jealousy or resentment. Added to these changes in the roles of each partner, the strains and pressures of an increasingly busy lifestyle, with longer hours, weekend work and fewer holidays to generate necessary income, can often cause practical problems in any relationship. When to see one another and relax can become a major issue; intimacy in the relationship can literally become difficult to maintain.

Married couples have traditionally had to show patience and commitment in order to maintain a healthy relationship. These days the number of divorces is massively on the increase and the ability to maintain a quality relationship over time seems harder than ever. Probably we are literally spoiled for choice, with growing evidence all round us that changing partners is as easy as changing your car. However, the need for intimacy is strong in all of us and this mostly occurs through touch, especially the kind of touch sanctioned within intimate relationships.

Interestingly, this may be more true of women, whose tactile needs are apparently greater than men's. Men are more visually stimulated, and this fact has perhaps allowed for many men to become more easily isolated sexually. Some may come to rely on pornography for self-gratification. In extreme cases they may turn to the perverted expression of their repressed sexual desires through sex crime.

Relationships, whether intimate or not, are clearly at the heart of being human. They are what motivate and excite, whether sexually or not. The challenge facing couples today is how to sustain a happy, fulfilled and exciting relationship and still meet the demands of an ever more busy lifestyle. Unfortunately, so many of the methods we use to cope with the daily strains of life — alcohol, stimulants like tea, coffee, cigarettes or drugs, even chocolate — all these have a disastrous effect on our libido and our general health, as does the direct effect of stress itself.

The most common complaint in the GP's surgery after cardiac problems is still tiredness and fatigue. How can we lead life to the full and still have enough in reserve for our partner? Certainly, relationships require energy and it is often energy which is lacking at the end of a long stressful day at work. Yet we owe it to ourselves to enjoy our relationships, to let intimate contact with another human being relax and recharge us as well as allow us to contribute to our partner. Finally, we owe it to a future generation. In Taoist sexual practice they say that the condition of the sperm and the ovum are adversely affected by poor health and negative emotions so that healthy children can only result from healthy relationships.

Shiatsu

Oriental massage of all kinds is based on harmonizing the body's energy system and restoring the proper flow of energy. It is excellent for combating fatigue and general energy loss. For couples, loss of sexual stamina is usually the first symptom of general loss of vitality and may lead to more severe sexual problems such as frigidity, impotence or premature ejaculation. Clearly, the psychological element of such disorders plays a large part too. But regular gentle, loving touch and affection, not necessarily sexually motivated, will often satisfy a person's emotional and psychological as well as physical needs. A good sex life often depends on our ability to feel relaxed and free from anxiety. When the muscles in our body are tense and inflexible, our sexual sensitivity is dulled. Areas which are particularly associated with sexual vigour are the back, especially the lower part, the abdomen and the legs.

In Oriental medicine, the bladder and kidney meridians are distributed in these areas and treatment of sexual problems is usually focused here. The concept of the kidney holds particular significance in Oriental medicine with regard to sexual vitality. It is seen as the organ which stores essence or vital energy, needed to sustain life. Traditionally, the Chinese believed that it is depleted in men through ejaculation and in women through childbirth. This accounts for much of Taoist sexual practice being centred on so-called 'internal orgasm' in men where semen is drawn back into the testes during orgasm and not lost, and very careful ante- and post-natal practices for women involving various diets, herbs and exercises. Since the Oriental concept of the kidney includes the adrenals, important areas to include for Shiatsu are the kidney area itself as well as points affecting the pituitary gland on the head and the thyroid gland on the neck. Again, these points will mostly be located along the kidney and bladder meridians.

Other meridians may also be involved in sexual problems. Where worry or anxiety are the main cause, the heart and small intestine meridian may be involved. In cases of impotence or premature ejaculation, the liver and gall bladder meridians are affected. Where general energy is lacking, poor diet and/or lack of exercise may be suspected and often the spleen (and pancreas) and stomach or the lung and large intestine meridians will be affected respectively. Points along these channels may also be used in shiatsu.

Finally, when practising a sequence of strokes, it is much more effective to begin with simple, soothing strokes (see page 60) to relax your partner before concentrating on the key areas for Shiatsu. It is essential to create a caring supportive atmosphere conducive to a sexual relationship to give you the best chance of success. Sexual energy is extremely subtle and capricious and will not simply respond to crude stimulation, at least not in a way that will ultimately support your health! Whilst people in later life may naturally experience a decline in sexual vitality, this should not affect the quality of their relationship or general health. Today, too many younger people, especially men, are experiencing sudden loss of sexual and overall vigour. Perhaps too much attention is focused on the attainment of pure sexual pleasure, whether through the obsessive nature of the individual or the pressures of a stressful, goal-oriented society. Shiatsu and massage work directly and indirectly to ease psychological and physical tension and can help build mutual trust and understanding between couples, helping them to develop the ability to cope with stressful situations and maintain good health.

Note: It should be mentioned that not all sexual problems are environmentally or psychologically induced. Couples should always check for physical abnormalities as a precaution.

Beginning sequences

For the beginning sequence it is better for the receiver to be naked and for the giver to use oils (see aromatherapy section).

1. Receiver lying on stomach. Giver kneeling above head facing feet. Smooth flowing palm stokes down back to buttocks and back up sides of back. This will relax your partner and unblock energy in the bladder meridian. (*figs. 62 and 63*)

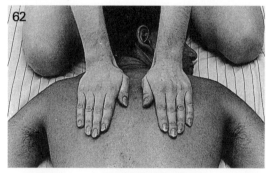

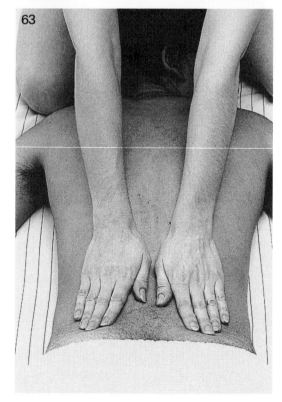

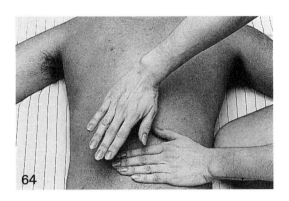

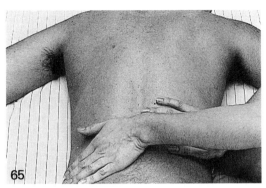

2. Receiver lying on stomach. Giver kneeling at side facing low back. Smooth clockwise movements of the palm over the kidney area. This is to harmonize kidney energy (*figs. 64 and 65*).

3. Receiver lying on back. Giver kneeling alongside facing head. Palming down to lower abdomen from under ribs (*fig. 66*). Left hand from right side, right hand from left side. Alternate hands using mainly fingers in smooth rhythmic action (*fig. 67*). This is to harmonize liver and spleen energy with the kidney.

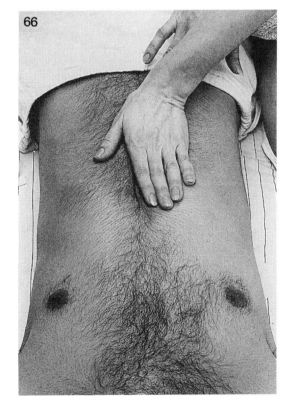

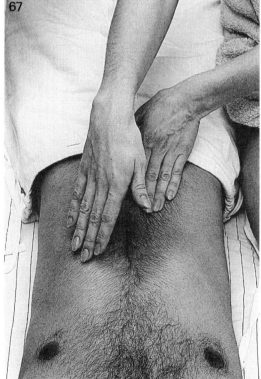

4. Same position for receiver, giver turns to face lower abdomen, kneeling. Smooth clockwise movements of the palm over the umbilical area and just below. (*figs. 68 and 69*). This is for harmonizing kidney energy.

5. Receiver remains on back, legs apart. Giver kneels between legs facing head, with partner's legs resting on knees (*fig. 70*). Smooth gentle stroking palm movements up inside of thighs from knees to groin (*fig. 71*), down outside of thighs back to knees (*fig. 72*). This will promote energy flow in the liver, spleen and especially kidney meridians.

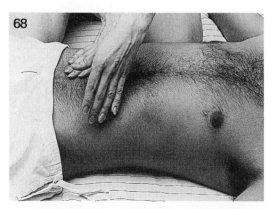

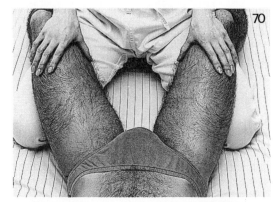

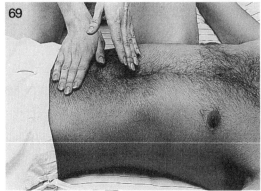

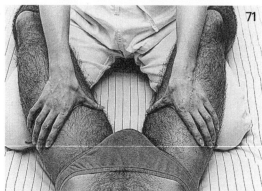

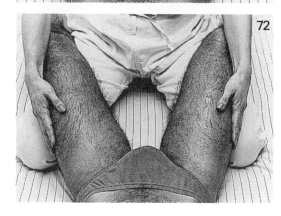

Shiatsu points

1. Receiver lying on stomach. Giver kneeling alongside back. Press bladder points UB 18 (*fig. 73*), UB 19 (*fig. 74*), UB 20 (*fig. 75*), UB 23 (*fig. 76*), UB 24 (*fig. 77*), UB 26 (*fig. 78*), with thumbs in pairs. Also GV 4 (*fig. 79*) — thumbs crossed.

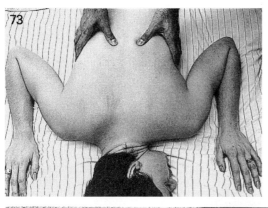

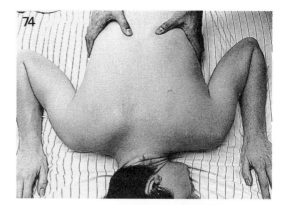

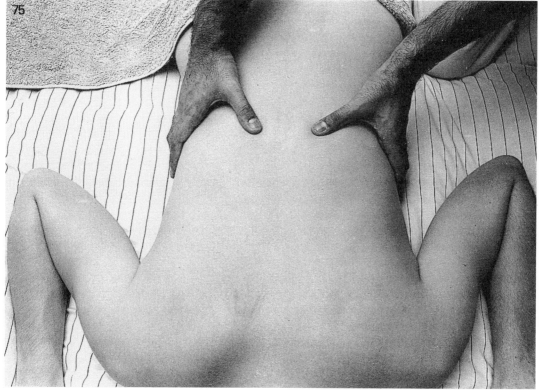

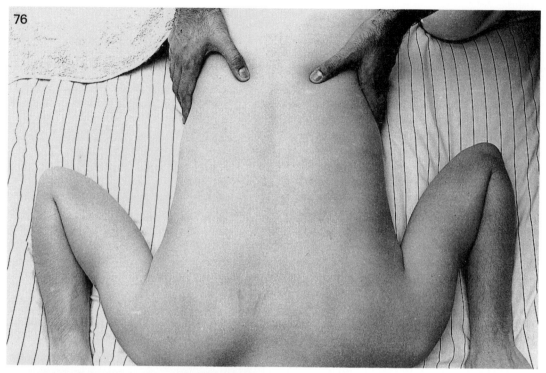

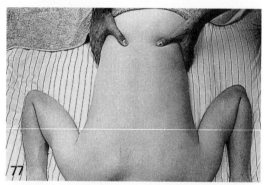

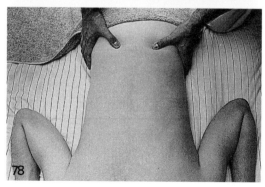

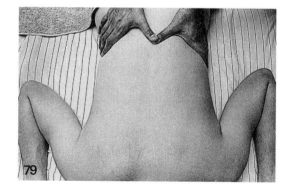

2. Move down level with buttocks. Outside leg raised (½ kneeling position). Press bladder points UB 28 (*fig. 80*), UB 31-34 (*fig. 81*) with thumbs in pairs. Then press down centre of sacrum from GV 3 (*fig. 82*), to GV 2 (*fig. 83*).

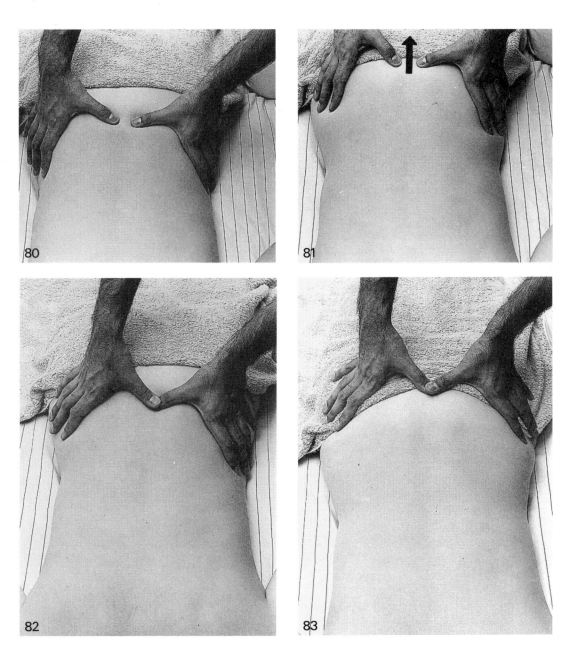

3. Receiver lying on back. Giver kneeling alongside abdomen. Press along kidney meridian from Ki 16 (*fig. 84*) to Ki 11 (*fig. 85*). Then press down midline of lower abdomen from CV 6 (*fig. 86*) to CV 2 (*fig. 87*). Also press Liv. 12 (*fig. 88*) and along groin area both sides.

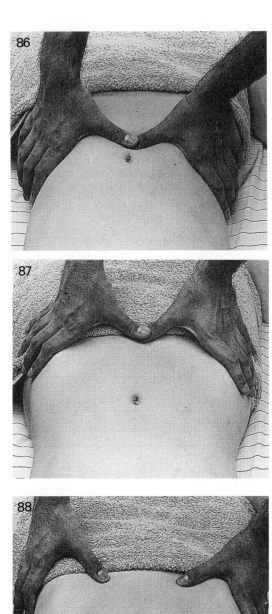

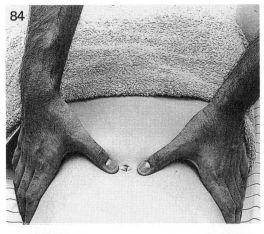

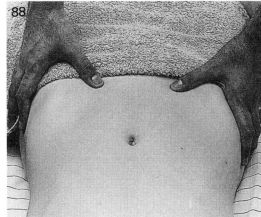

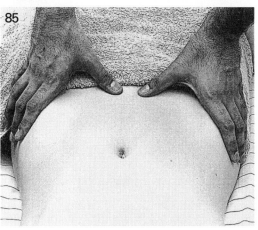

4. Receiver raises legs and opens them apart. Giver applies pressure at point CV 1 (*fig. 88a*) firmly. This is good for immediate stimulation of the sexual organs.

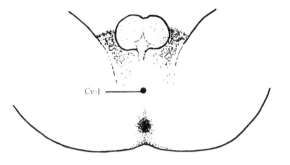

5. Giver moves to legs. Press points St 36 (*fig. 89*), Sp 6 (*fig. 90*), Ki (*fig. 91*). On the feet press points in arch of foot around Ki 2 (*fig. 92*) and on the sole, concentrate on Ki 1 (*fig. 93*). (You may also walk on your partner's feet.) This point will usually be sore in sexual problems and is very effective.

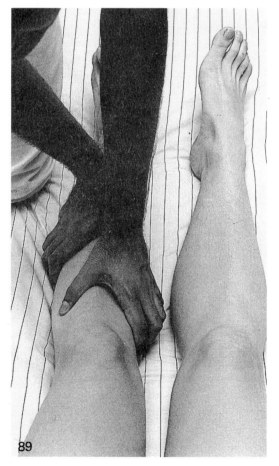

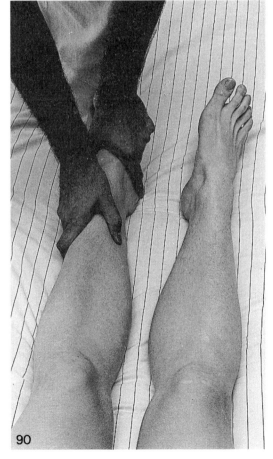

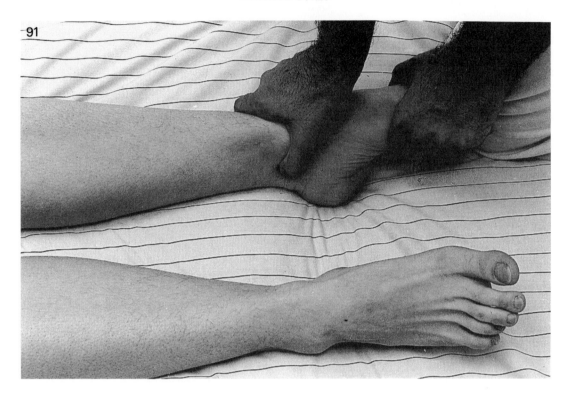

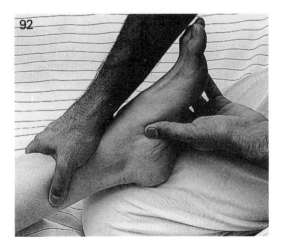

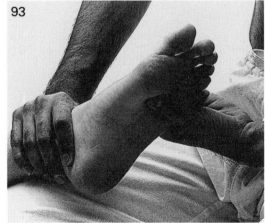

6. Finally move to the head. Press points on either side of front of neck around St 9 (*fig. 94*). Press GV 20 (*fig. 95*).

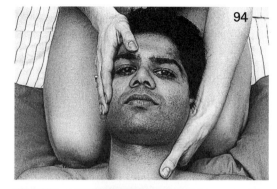

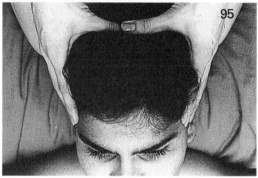

Exercise

Many relationship problems involving tension and loss of vitality and sexual desire may simply be the result of lack of exercise. The importance of exercise in maintaining general health is discussed in Chapter 10, but its connection with sexual vitality is obvious. We have seen how exercise can uplift you and give you an emotional 'high' as well as the physical benefits of cardiovascular fitness, improved internal secretions and general body relaxation and muscle tonus. All of these things will contribute to a healthy relationship. External exercise will improve stamina and sexual performance, though too much overtly physical exercise may be counterproductive. Internal exercise is probably the most effective way to enhance vitality and is centred on cultivating and improving the flow of energy throughout the body. Taoist sexual practice, chi-kung and Do-in ankyo are some of the systems drawn from here to suggest ways of cultivating our sexual vitality. These are especially applicable to men. See Bibliography for books on these subjects.

Sexual problems

Below are a number of common problems, both psychological and sexual, which may inhibit a harmonious loving relationship. Poor communication is the fundamental cause underlying the majority of relationship and sexual difficulties.

The lasting solution therefore is to improve communication and understanding between yourself and your partner. The value of massage is unequalled in this respect for it allows us to convey and share loving intimacy without the necessity of sex. Often, lovemaking can become predictable and perfunctory and this can lead to boredom and dissatisfaction within the relationship as a whole.

Massage presents the opportunity to convey affection, love and pleasure in a way that is totally giving with your partner not needing or having to do anything in return. Massage can be an extraordinary experience of total giving or receiving. In recommending massage we also recommend that you do not necessarily see it as a prerequisite or automatic lead into sexual intercourse. This may well be the case but the intention should be to give unconditionally without an effect or result in mind.

Massage will give you a new understanding of your lover's body. You will become newly acquainted with the fine details of their unique physical characteristics. You will become finely tuned at what feels particularly pleasant or ticklish or uncomfortable for your partner's body. We often limit ourselves by seeing only the genitals as being erotic.

However, the ears, hands, feet, solar plexus, back of the knees, and the back of the neck are all erogenous zones. These areas house nerve endings and are linked to hormone-producing glands. Stimulation of these areas can create sexual desire and long-term drive. Massage is also the ideal way to provide for the smooth transition between our everyday activities and business to the quieter mode necessary for relaxation and quality time together. A short neck and shoulders treatment from your partner will be much more beneficial and enjoyable than the typical cigarette and gin and tonic. (See Chapter 3 for sequences.) Massage is also perfect for older couples who may not include sexual intercourse so much within their relationship. Massage encourages them to stay in touch and express their affection in an intimate physical manner.

Loss of libido

The sense of smell has a powerful effect on our emotions and our passions. The perfume and cosmetic industry is only too well aware of this and make vast profits out of our sense of smell. We may even be largely unaware of this, but our senses will be attracted or repelled by certain smells. Fragrance can inspire romance and sexual passion. Natural scents are the most erotic: Patchouli, Ylang-ylang and Jasmine are renowned for their erotic power. All of the oils are relaxing and soothing by nature, so will alleviate the underlying cause of frigidity and low libido, which is usually mental and emotional tension and stress. The oils are best used as part of a massage treatment by one lover to another and can also be used as a relaxing night-time bath treatment. Finally, it should be remembered that sexual problems are most usually a reflection of a lack of closeness within the relationship. With the increasing demands on our time and energy, it is essential to plan for quality time for your relationship to develop and grow. You may actually need to book time into your week when you will spend time together for recreational and social activities and for quiet intimate time together. Your relationship is like a delicate flower: if you nourish it, it will enhance your life and give you great pleasure. If you take it for granted and ignore it, it will dry up and die.

Massage also increases our personal self-esteem so we are more at ease with our bodies. Rose, Neroli, Clary sage, Patchouli, Ylang-ylang, Jasmine and Sandalwood: choose the oils you find most appealing and combine up to three in a massage oil or in a bath.

Tiredness

Use Rosemary or Bergamot oil in baths and for massage and handkerchief inhalation.

AIDS

All the sexually-transmitted diseases and AIDS have one thing in common. They can all come about and take hold in the body when the immune system is weakened. AIDS requires complex treatment, but there are oils which do have a strengthening effect on the immune system. There is increasing evidence from the USA that natural therapies such as nutrition, acupuncture, herbalism, massage, aromatherapy and attitudinal change can help prevent the onset of full-blown AIDS, increase periods of remission and even lead to a better quality of life.

In a relationship where one partner has AIDS, massage is a wonderful way to retain physical love and intimacy without any danger of infection. A life-threatening illness like AIDS can be extremely distressing and isolating. Loving, caring touch is more essential than ever to convey reassurance and acceptance. The following oils can be used in massage or as a bath treatment, though any of them are useful for sexually-transmitted diseases and AIDS: Lavender, Bergamot, Eucalyptus, Rosemary, Geranium and Tea tree.

Stress, tension and anxiety

The oils are ideal for the treatment of these conditions since they all have the inherent properties to calm, relax and uplift at the same time. The best way to use the oils is through massage, as it is the caring touch of the giver which will ease and release worry and induce feelings of calm and relaxation.

The following oils may be used in a massage oil or in the bath, with a combination of no more than three: Bergamot, Geranium, Lavender, Camomile, Ylang-ylang, Neroli, Rose and Marjoram. As always, use your friend's preference as your guideline in your choice of three oils.

Self-esteem

The importance and value of individual self-esteem within a relationship are great. If we feel good about our physical appearance, we are much more likely to enjoy and take pleasure in our bodies. If we feel that we deserve to have our needs met, we will ask for and most likely receive what we want. The following affirmations will assist you in feeling better about yourself, your body and your worth as an individual. A powerful and fun way to use these high quality thoughts is to whisper and say them to each other as you go to sleep!

○ I, (insert your name), can say 'no' without losing my partner's love.
○ I am good enough as a woman/man.
○ I . . . am a beautiful woman/man and I deserve to be loved.
○ I . . . am now asking for what I want and having my needs met.
○ I . . . have a beautiful body and I enjoy taking care of it.
○ I . . . am now loving my body and giving it the very best.
○ I . . . now tell the truth and express my feelings honestly.
○ Because I . . . am good enough, I can relax and enjoy my sexuality.
○ I . . . am good enough at everything I do.
○ I . . . have an attractive, strong body which is worthy of love.

5

Menstruation and menopause

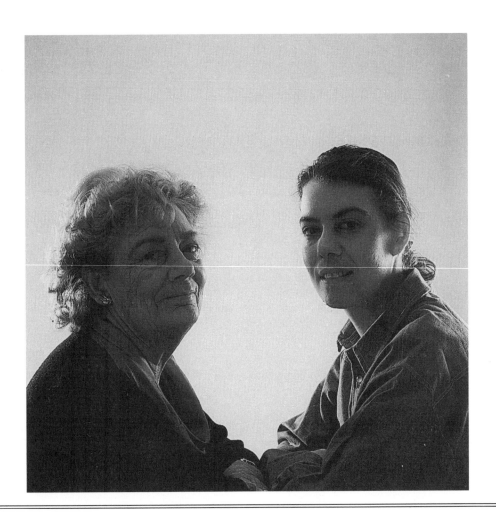

Menstruation is a periodic change common to the females of the higher apes as well as to humans. It involves the flow of blood from the womb in regular, monthly cycles starting from the age of 12–16 years and continuing until about age 45 or 50. Its onset is associated with puberty. The start is called the menarche and the end is at the menopause. The term menopause describes the cessation of menstruation and marks the end of reproductive life. There is considerable variation in time of onset, cycle and cessation according to geography, race, climate, diet and emotional and physical states.

In ancient Greece the body was believed to renew itself every seven years, and the numerological significance of seven is well-known in the East. The Chinese observed clear physical and psychological transformations at multiples of seven years throughout life. The Nei Ching states: 'When a girl is seven years of age . . . she begins to change her teeth and her hair grows longer. When she reaches her fourteenth year she begins to menstruate and is able to become pregnant . . . when the girl reaches the age of 21 years . . . the last tooth has come out and she is fully grown. When she reaches the age of 49 she can no longer become pregnant . . . her menstruation is exhausted . . . and she is no longer able to bear children.'

Though written more than 2,000 years ago, this is a pretty accurate description of the growth and development of the woman from puberty to menopause. The word climacteric is often used to mark the passage of such stages in a person's life, heralding major change. It is an appropriate word with an obvious link to the seasonal and climatic influences which we all, especially women, link to the functioning of our bodies. Women in many societies would acknowledge the effect of the moon on their menstrual cycle. In ancient cultures such as the Chinese, it was thought natural that the woman would menstruate at the time of the full moon. In the Nei Ching it says that 'When the moon is full to the rim there is abundance of blood. . .'

Astrologers would attribute the influence of the planets to such climacterics just the same way. Historically at least, menstruation and menopause are seen as natural phenomena inextricably linked with the influence of certain cosmic forces yet fundamentally and integrally part of the physiology of women. In fact, many tribal cultures have elaborate rituals to prepare for and celebrate the onset of puberty as well as the passing of fertility.

This is in stark contrast to many of the taboos that have grown up around these subjects in Western society. The concept of the 'curse', derived from God's punishment to Eve in the Old Testament, still permeates much of our thinking. Menstruation has come to be seen as a regular nuisance, carrying countless euphemisms which suggest that many women still see it as a burden, and often one they deserve and must endure. Similarly, menopause for the same women has become the convenient excuse for a whole host of mid-life crises, both physical and emotional. Women have almost come to expect that they will feel irrational, moody and generally out of sorts for anything between one and five years.

For such a huge feature, little attention is paid either to its onset or the changes it brings with it every month. This is due to the mystery and silence that still surrounds menstruation for young women.

One effect of this lack of acceptance and appreciation of menstruation is the widespread ignorance expressed by women towards this biological event. This ignorance is often passed down from mother to daughter, so we often see the daughter, as a young woman of 12 or 13, beginning to menstruate with no real knowledge of the monthly effects of this major event. This ignorance has far-reaching repercussions. We are at the mercy of what we don't understand, which means we are also powerless to shape the impact of it on our lives. The young woman coming to adolescence has no tools for gaining insight and self-awareness. Menstruation can be held responsible for an overall feeling of lack of control over her body, her moods and herself; leaving her feeling insecure and unable to trust or rely on herself.

It is in this context that women experience menstruation. No wonder that they often feel unable to cope with this process. We are clearly out of touch with the changes that take place within our bodies as a result of the hormonal cycle. We largely experience variation in moods and energy levels as a regular but arbitrary part of life. We are also out of touch with our body's nutritional needs. Premenstrual syndrome and many of its consequences have recently been treated with great success by improvements in nutrition and diet. This works especially well in the area of water retention and its attendant weight gain and mood swings.

A failure to fully comprehend the function of menstruation and menopause within the natural process of maturing and developing may lie at the root of many things we conceive of as 'problems'. Many women in today's society easily become out of touch with their bodies and seek only to suppress any painful or unpleasant experiences associated with them. Massage therapy is a perfect way to stay in touch with our body and learn to gain distinctions for ourselves in judging what is and what is not a natural experience. Ideally, menstruation would start smoothly and painlessly and continue with ease and regularity throughout life. Cessation at menopause would occur equally effortlessly and with no major physical or psychological upset.

Unfortunately, today's lifestyle allows for many attitude influences to affect such a smooth flow of events. Stimulants like cigarettes, coffee, even drugs or depressants like alcohol; stress, both physical and emotional; irregular or poor diet; lack of exercise and sleep; and, not least, various methods of birth control, most obviously the pill — all have taken their toll in interrupting a woman's natural cycle.

Premenstrual tension (PMT), irregular menstruation, including amenorrhoea (lack of menstruation) and dysmenorrhoea (heavy period pain): what is for some cultures a joyous celebration of womanhood has become, literally, a curse to be put up with and where possible avoided completely.

One thing is clear. The onset and cessation of a woman's period (the menarche and menopause), as well as continued menstruation during the period in between, all require a woman to adapt to great changes in her bodily and mental functions. Fine chemical adjustments are being made at these times in the diencephalon, the area between the left and right lobes of the brain, affecting the pituitary gland and the release of sex hormones. Emotional upset, sudden shocks, weather changes, poor sleep and diet, overstrain and stress can all influence this process of adaptation and lead to symptoms of disorientation and imbalance. Most common are hot flushes, headaches, palpitations, nervous irritability, depression and general debility as well as possible weight gain or loss.

Care should be taken at these times to get medical advice to distinguish such hormonal imbalances from other more serious disorders. Sometimes there may be a tendency to dismiss such symptoms as being part of a particular stage of a woman's development: 'She's coming of age. . .'; 'it's her time of the month' or the very frequent 'it must be the menopause.' In reality, it is always worth checking for other gynaecological complications or metabolic dysfunctions such as thyroid problems, as well as psychological disorders. Otherwise, such climacteric changes in a woman's life may often be dealt with by proper diet, regular exercise, good sleep and relaxation as well as by some of the simple suggestions listed below.

It should be noted that interference with

the natural changes occurring in the body at puberty and at the time of the menopause are best treated naturally. The least intervention possible is recommended. Treatments such as the pill for young girls experiencing painful onset of menstruation or the now-common hormone replacement treatment, while they may alleviate some symptoms, generally retard the whole process of adaptation and adjustment. They may also produce unpleasant side-effects.

With greater understanding and appreciation we would also be in a position to exploit the variations in our distinct energy levels during the monthly cycle. For example, the week prior to menstruation is a time when most women experience intense tiredness and a desire to sleep and daydream. This could be seen as a great nuisance and interruption to our busy inflexible routine or as an opportunity to gain greater insight and understanding of ourselves and our subconscious. We are normally quite out of touch with our subconscious, and access to it provides profound inspiration and creative thought. We could prioritize this time for inner reflection and caring, and nurturing of ourselves; taking time to be deeply in contact with ourselves and our needs. Recharging our energy in this way prepares us for the active time, during mid-cycle, when our energy is more outgoing and vigorous. Menstruation could become a reliable method of planning the best times for particular events in our routine: allowing for the dynamic ebb and flow of our energy throughout the month.

In the East this appreciation of rhythm — highs and lows and ebb and flow of life — is intrinsic to their philosophy and permeates their medical system. The flowing of the seasons is understood to have its effect on the human body and psyche and throughout the natural world. The Japanese chart the individual biorhythms of their employees to obtain precise information regarding their energy levels. With this information employees are given days off when their energy suggests they would be accident-prone or generally sluggish. Since Japan is an extremely powerful industrial nation, we have a great deal to learn from the Japanese. With this simple device, the rate of accidents at work has been substantially decreased, as have days lost through sickness.

Biorhythms, the rhythm of energy, could well be the hormonal equivalent of menstruation for men. Clearly our energy does fluctuate and vary: and to take full benefit of this natural flow we need to have tools with which to understand the process. Simple information and a more enlightened attitude to menstruation could transform it to enhance our well-being and quality of life. The time may well come when both men and women have 'time out' when their individual rhythms and cycles point towards rest and recuperation, and work when their energy is vigorous and strong. We could then always be aligned to our particular activity at any time.

Massage and Shiatsu

Menstruation

A woman who experiences menstruation problems will generally hold tension in her low-back region and over the sacrum, in the lower abdomen and often in the neck and shoulders. However, since every woman experiences menstruation differently, each may have particular areas of tension or discomfort associated with her period, and this must be located. For pain or dysmenorrhoea, local massaging and shiatsu are more effective when done in the premenstrual phase and not during menstruation itself when it is likely to be less effective and even painful. The aim is to regulate hormone production and distribution, strengthen the uterus, move and circulate the blood, revitalize stagnant body energy and balance the whole person.

You may use the neck and shoulder treatment described in Chapter 3. Pay particular attention to the occipital region and give firm, sustained pressure to point GV 15, at the nape of the neck (where the spinal cord projects into the brain; page 185). This stimulates hormone secretion. For the low-back and sacrum use the sequence described in Chapter 4 and especially concentrate on the following points: UB 22/23 which control whole body energy, both essential and acquired (UB 23 also regulates kidney function); UB 18/20 to stimulate liver and spleen functions, regulating the production and distribution of blood; UB 31/32/33/34 which affect the urogenital organs directly.

Buttock massage is also appropriate here as well as massage all over the sacrum. Abdominal massage is highly effective for menstrual problems but must be done gently and carefully. It is best avoided once menstruation has begun or when there is severe cramping.

Receiver lies comfortably on her back, knees up where necessary. Sit alongside receiver and gently stroke up, down, lengthways and in circles.

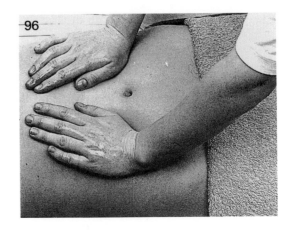

Massage — Ampuku After massaging and relaxing the whole area (*figs. 96 and 97*) concentrate on pressure with crossed thumbs on the following points.

Note: You should give firm pressure at first, then, when you feel the abdomen relax, go deeper. Hold the point until you feel it 'fill up' and gradually release it on every in breath of the receiver until skin contact is broken, then move on.

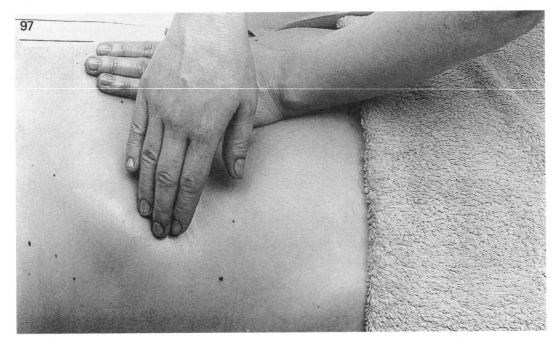

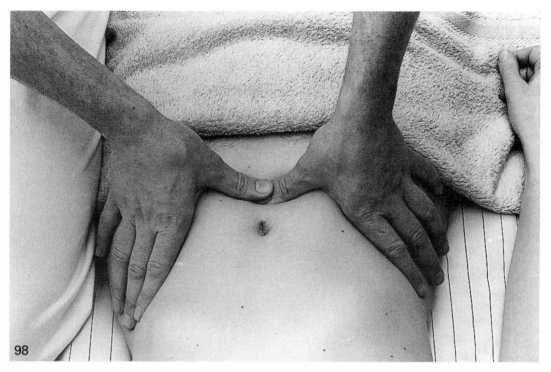

CV 6 (*fig. 98*), CV 4 (*fig. 99*) for general vitality and stimulation of kidney function, respectively.

CV 3 (*fig. 100*), Ki 12 (*fig. 101*) and points

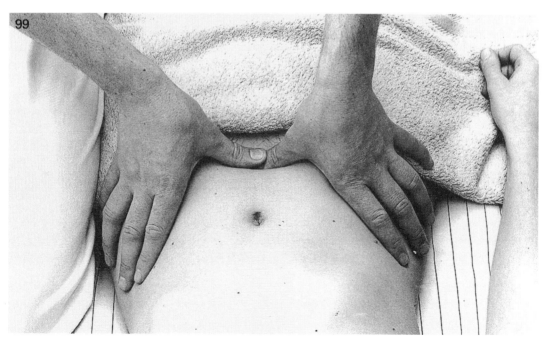

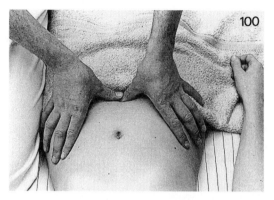

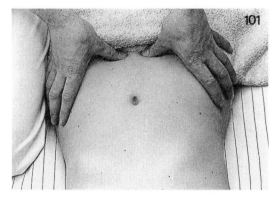

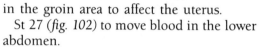

in the groin area to affect the uterus.

St 27 (*fig. 102*) to move blood in the lower abdomen.

Finally, the inside of the legs are often used to regulate menstruation, not only to increase circulation and draw obstruction away from the abdominal region, but also because of the location of key meridians in this area. These are mainly for liver, responsible in Chinese medicine for distribution of blood; the spleen, responsible for blood production and the kidney, contributing to blood production and controlling fluid secretion (including hormones).

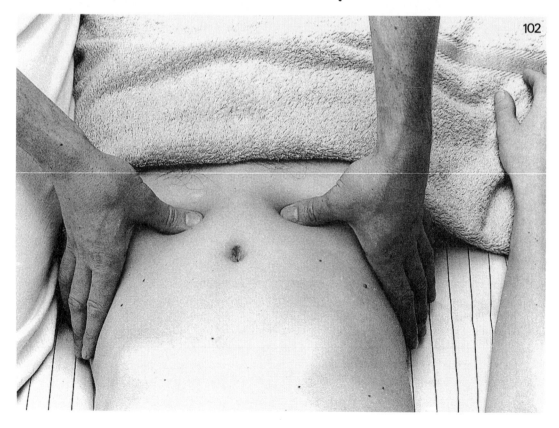

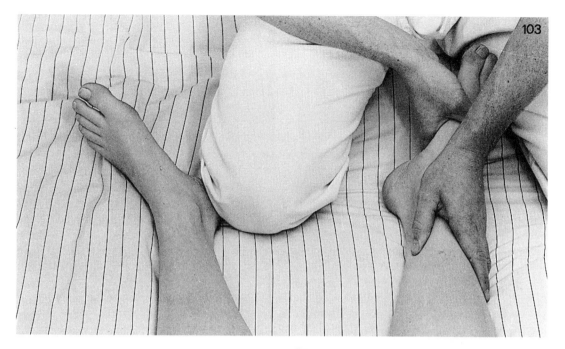

Use a general massage sequence — see pages 172-5) concentrating on the following points: Sp 6 (*fig. 103*), Sp 10 (*fig. 104*): regulation of menses and blood production.

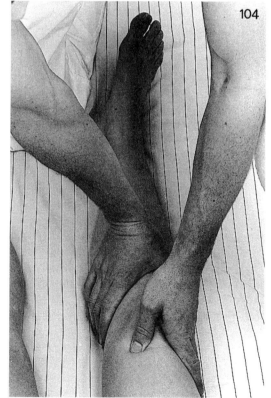

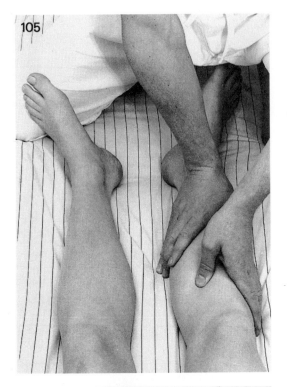

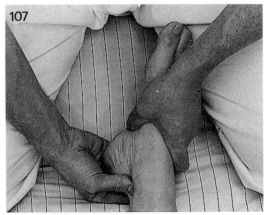

Sp 8 (*fig. 105*): painful menstruation.
Sp 9 (*fig. 106*), Ki 3 (*fig. 107*), Ki 7, (*fig. 108*): internal secretions and water retention.

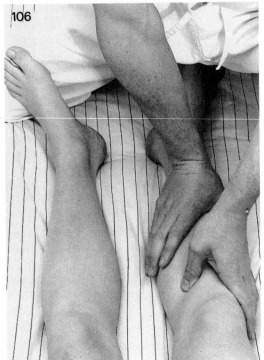

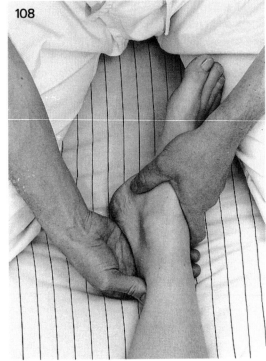

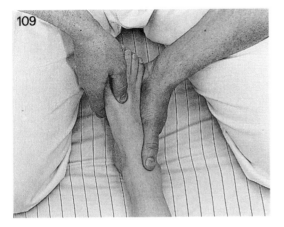

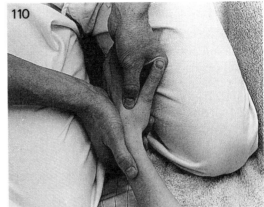

Liv 3 (*fig. 109*) and LI 4 (*fig. 110*) combined can be used to regulate blood and energy flow in the whole body and will reduce painful menstruation, as well as any headaches associated with it.

Painful periods can often be caused or exacerbated by the cold. Some women use hot water bottles to ease discomfort. Moxibustion, the burning of a medicinal herb on or near the skin, is extremely useful for severe, contracting cramps and pains during menstruation. Use the abdominal and leg points.

Menopause

General, whole body massage and Shiatsu is recommended regularly throughout the period of the menopause to help the body readjust to hormonal and other changes. As in the menstruation section above, areas to concentrate on include the low-back and sacrum, as well as the back of the head, neck and shoulders.

The use of points is also similar and all of the points above may be used, though Sp 6, UB10, 23, Ki 3, Liv 3 and LI 4 may usefully deal with some specific symptoms like headaches, flushes, constipation etc. If emotional symptoms occur involving nervous irritability, anxiety and insomnia, points on the Ht and Pe meridians may be used especially Ht 7 (*fig. 111*). It should be noted that generally moxa is not used as many women experience hot flushes, and heat may aggravate these.

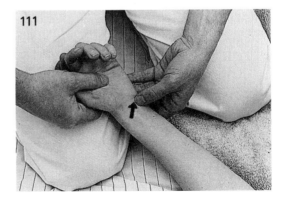

Exercise

All exercise should be directed at increasing circulation and thus exercises for cardiovascular fitness are recommended. Of the usual ones, swimming is recommended for the supportive quality of the water, with little compression or vibration of the lower abdomen.

Internal exercise should be directed at moving and circulating the energy and blood around the abdominal cavity and distributing it to the extremities. 'Hara' or belly breathing is recommended and can be practised whilst carrying out daily exercises like yoga or Tai Chi.

Bach remedies — menstruation

Feeling grubby, not fully accepting one's bodily changes:	Crab Apple
Lack of confidence, feeling unsure of oneself:	Larch
Impatience, irritability:	Impatiens
Worry, anxiety:	White Chestnut
Exhaustion, tiredness:	Olive
Emergency combination remedy for extreme distress:	Rescue remedy

Menopause
Same as for above except for:

Adjustment to change, transition:	Walnut

Oils

The oils can be of great benefit for all problems associated with menopause. As with most other problems they are best used with massage. However, any prolonged difficulties or severe pain should be checked by a gynaecologist to be fully sure you are not missing a medical condition that needs treatment.

Painful periods, sharp piercing pain: Lavender, Marjoram.

Dull ache: Camomile, Marjoram. Use in massage to work gently over the stomach and lower back or in a hot compress.

Fluid retention: Geranium, Rose. Use in massage and baths.

Depression and irritability: Bergamot, Camomile, Rose, Melissa. Use in massage, baths, handkerchief inhalation.

Irregular periods, excessively heavy periods: Cypress, Geranium, Rose.

Menopause During menopause, each woman's experience and symptoms all vary. But we can categorize some of the most common:

Depression, anxiety, worry: Bergamot, Melissa, Lavender, Neroli, Ylang-ylang, Jasmine.

Mood swings: Geranium, Rose, Camomile.

All the above oils can be used in a combination of massage, baths and handkerchief inhalation.

Self-esteem

Menstruation
- It's OK and safe for me to relax.
- I, . . ., am relaxed in whatever I'm doing.
- I, . . ., love and accept my body completely.
- I, . . ., accept myself as a woman and enjoy my body's natural rhythms.
- I love and approve of myself.

Louise Hay, in her book *You Can Heal Your Life*, has some interesting thoughts to offer relating to specific ailments:

Ailment	Probable cause	New thought
Cramps	Tension, fear gripping, holding on.	I relax and allow my mind to be peaceful.
Menstrual problems	Rejection of one's femininity. Guilt, fear.	I accept my full power as a woman and accept all my bodily processes as normal. I love and approve of myself.
Premenstrual syndrome	Allowing confusion to reign. Giving power to outside influences. Rejection of the feminine processes.	I now take charge of my mind, and my life. I am a powerful, dynamite woman! Every part of my body functions perfectly. I love me.

Menopause

For menopause Louise Hay recommends the following:

Menopause	Fear of no longer being wanted. Fear of ageing. Self-rejection. Not being good enough.	I am balanced and peaceful in all changes of cycles and I bless my body with love.
Fatigue	Resistance, boredom. Lacking love for what one does.	I am enthusiastic about life and filled with energy and enthusiasm.

Other thoughts that will prove supportive are: I am good enough as a woman. I am a beautiful, sensual woman and I deserve to be loved. My life is wonderful and my future full of terrific surprises. I love and approve of myself completely.

Abdominal massage

This is a particularly sensitive area of the body, especially prior to and during menstruation. Your touch should therefore be firm and reassuringly slow. If you are just working on the abdomen, cover the upper chest area with a towel and make sure your partner is warm enough.

1) Kneel alongside your partner, take her arm out to the side and very slowly make contact.

2) Apply the oil to your hands and begin to effleurage the belly. Begin with both hands above the navel, stroke up to ribcage, down sides of torso, on to lower abdomen and glide up to navel. Repeat slowly at least ten times.

3) Rest one hand on near side of belly and with the other make clockwise circles on the belly.

4) Knead entire area including sides of torso gently.

5) Repeat effleurage slowly at least three times.

6

Pregnancy and childbirth

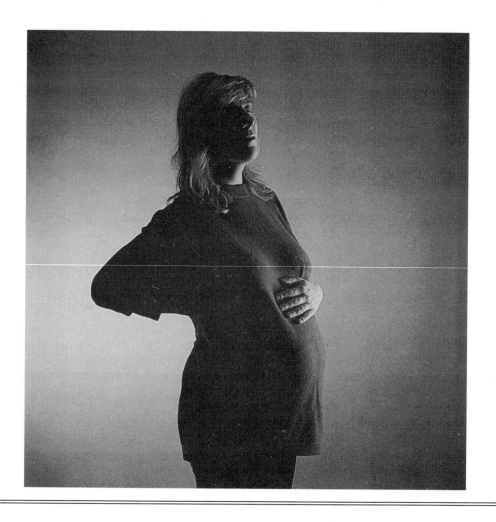

Pregnancy is a time of great change and transition for a woman and her body. In the short space of nine months, her body will progress from conception to having a fully formed human being (albeit a small one!) in her womb.

It is a time filled with rapid physical adjustments and emotional extremes. These can include unpleasant or distressing physical symptoms such as morning sickness, headaches, constipation, muscle cramps, backache, heartburn, indigestion, varicosities and fatigue, or the familiar moodiness and depression which can accompany pregnancy and especially after the birth itself.

A woman may experience extreme mood changes along with extreme physical change. Handling these changes and the attendant problems they may bring will promote a happy pregnancy, happy mother and trouble-free birth. The Active Birth movement of the early 1980s spearheaded a radical new attitude to childbearing: putting the woman in a much more active role both during pregnancy and childbirth. The natural birth movement, like the natural health movement, has emphasized the need to take responsibility for our health, pregnancy and the act of giving birth. Large numbers of woman are no longer content to remain ignorant and passive during their pregnancy and then have the birth managed by experts in hospital. Since 1982, when the Active Birth Manifesto was declared and published, many women have chosen to have their babies at home. Increasing numbers of hospitals are allowing women to choose to have their baby at home.

In taking responsibility for our health during pregnancy, we need to be as informed as possible in order to understand as fully as possible, and to flow with the rapid physical and hormonal changes taking place. With information at our fingertips we are then in a position to play a leading role in one of the most major events of our lives.

Taking care of ourselves is even made neces-sary by the contraindications of most drugs. Taking our ailment to our GP will probably only ever elicit sympathy, with advice to take it easy and rest. For some of the complaints associated with pregnancy, rest and endurance may be the only remedy. For example, it is common to experience extreme fatigue in the first three months of pregnancy. It is simply the body's way of ensuring adequate rest to allow for the rapid growing of the baby at this stage. It is helpful to acknowledge this and enjoy the dreaminess and pleasure that rest can bring.

A unique bridge

Pregnancy can often put added strain on a relationship at the very time when a loving, supportive partner is most needed. Some men become impatient, distant or just plain scared by an experience they find hard to understand. Sexual relationships may often be reduced or completely suppressed during pregnancy and this is a source of added frustration for the man. In the later stages of pregnancy both men and women may find it difficult to adjust to a new and often alarming body image, so often labelled ugly and unpleasant by many people. Massage provides a unique bridge between the partners at this challenging time, allowing them to give pleasure to and receive pleasure from one another in a nurturing, unselfish way without expectation.

Touch is the most direct bond we can experience and in massaging his expectant partner, a man may learn to relax her body in a totally new way. This is often sensual rather than sexual and allows for both partners to accept the new body as it is throughout the physical changes of pregnancy. Through touching and massage the couple are able to rediscover the beauty of pregnancy as a direct contact experience with a new life, created by them, rather than as an unpleasant image in their minds. This is a natural practice that will often carry over into later life and affect the quality and amount of touch within the family as a whole.

Because of the pressure exerted by the growing foetus (both back against the spine and, as it becomes heavier, down on the pelvis and legs), the last few months of pregnancy can often bring back pain, cramps and varicose veins in the legs, and fatigue. Massage is effective in relieving these problems by increasing circulation and relaxing the muscles. Following the birth, massage is useful in preventing stretchmarks of the breasts and abdomen by encouraging the muscles to tighten again.

At a time when most forms of internal medicine are contraindicated (even herbs), massage provides one of the main safe and totally natural ways to alleviate common symptoms and promote healthy pregnancy.

It is all too easy to focus on complaints and ailments during this time. However, it is also a rare and extraordinary time in which to develop a sixth sense and intuition regarding our bodies and their needs. It is an opportunity to be fully responsible for our health and know every decision we make regarding it has an effect and makes a difference to someone other than ourselves. It is a time to ask for support, delve into our feelings and fully enjoy the attention that the pregnant mother deserves. It is a time, more than any other, to prioritize our health, well-being and happiness; nine months in which to look after ourselves and be looked after like no other time before. Preparing for and giving birth to new life is surely one of the most important contributions we can ever make in the world. When we take responsibility for our health we are directly affecting the quality of life of another human being and another generation. A healthy, happy pregnancy is more likely to lead to a happy birth and baby and a more peaceful future.

Bach flower remedies

Transition, accepting change:	Walnut
Feeling ugly, unattractive:	Crab apple
Extreme tiredness:	Olive
Feeling resentful and put upon:	Willow
Not requesting adequate support:	Centaury
Gloom, doom, mood of depression descending for no reason:	Mustard
Impatience, irritability:	Impatiens
Fearful re the birth and the baby:	Aspen
Not able to take adequate rest, insisting on doing everything else first:	Rock water
Despondency, lack of enthusiasm:	Gentian
Distress/fear during the birth and afterwards:	Rescue remedy

Essential oils

Firstly, it is important to name the oils that must **not** be used during pregnancy: Basil, Camphor, Caraway, Clary sage, Cypress, Camomile, Cinammon, Fennel, Frankincense, Hyssop, Jasmine, Juniper, Marjoram, Myrrh, Peppermint, Pennyroyal, Rosemary, Sage, Thyme and Wintergreen.

Morning sickness/Nausea: Fennel tea — though not Fennel oil.

Backache: Lavender — in low dilution. In massage use only half the amount you normally would, that is, five drops to 20 ml vegetable oil. In baths — no more than four drops.

Fluid retention/oedema of the ankles and legs: Only include Rosemary from the sixth month onwards when the baby is fairly well established.

Massage and baths

Prevention of stretchmarks: Neroli; Mandarin. Massage the belly and hips with vegetable oil that includes 30 per cent wheatgerm oil.

Depression, anxiety: Rose, Bergamot, Neroli, Mandarin. (Massage; baths; handkerchief inhalations.)

During labour: Rose is reputed to strengthen contractions. Massage on the lower back during labour.

Postnatal depression: Rose, Melissa, Bergamot, Neroli, Geranium, Rosemary. (Massage; baths; handkerchief inhalations.)

Childbirth

Lavender and Jasmine are the two oils of most benefit during childbirth, as they strengthen and deepen contractions. Both oils can be used in the bath before and during labour. The oils can also be used in massage on the lower back, when the woman feels it would be helpful. Both oils have quite distinct aromas so the choice of oil to use would depend on the mother's preference.

Self-esteem

○ I now ask for support and am happy to receive it.
○ I now love and accept my body completely, however it looks.
○ I now vibrate with glowing health and energy.
○ I enjoy nourishing myself and giving my body the very best.

○ It's safe for me to trust the process of my body.
○ I look forward to my baby's birth with joy and excitement.

Massage

Early pregnancy: morning sickness; constipation and diarrhoea; fatigue; headaches and dizziness.
Later pregnancy: backache; circulatory problems including varicose veins and cramps; indigestion and heartburn.

Any of the above symptoms can occur at any time. The main difference in massage techniques is that in later pregnancy the woman may be limited to lying on her side or sitting down, facing the back of a chair. Generally, pressure must always be gentle and special care must be taken when massaging the lower back and abdomen. Women with weak constitutions or who have previously miscarried may need specialist attention and massage may be contraindicated, especially in the first three months. Complications such as anaemia, high blood pressure and malposition of the foetus will also need specialist attention. Massage should only be given with medical consent. In combination with regular exercise and good diet however, massage can help avoid and alleviate most of the common symptoms associated with pregnancy.

Sequences — back

Working on the back is a great stress reliever. It relaxes some of the largest muscles in the body. These become especially tense in later pregnancy as the baby becomes heavier and the mother's spine is distorted. Massage will reduce backache and promote healthy circulation in the uterus. In Chinese medicine the lower back, especially the sacrum, is closely linked with the urogenital function as well as with the uterus.

Note: In early pregnancy, the receiver may lie on her stomach but later on she may have only two positions to choose from for a back massage: 1) Receiver sits astride a chair using cushion to fully support abdomen. 2) Receiver lies on her side, upper knee bent and resting on pillow, head well supported on pillow.

Sitting position

1) Kneel behind partner.

2) Make contact on lower back.

3) Bring one foot up and effleurage leaning into back, up and around shoulders and down again. Use light pressure on lower back during first three months of pregnancy (*fig. 112*).

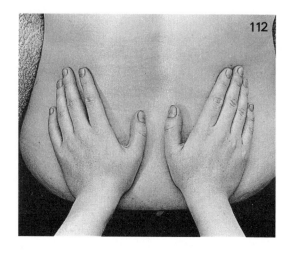

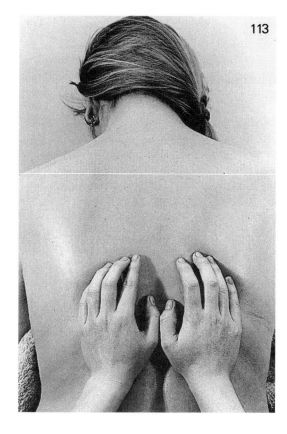

4) Lean heels of palms, whole hand in contact, into spine from sacrum to occiput (*fig. 113*).

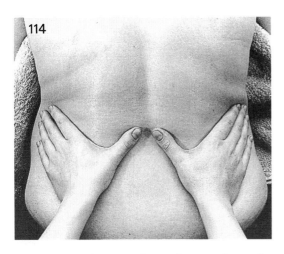

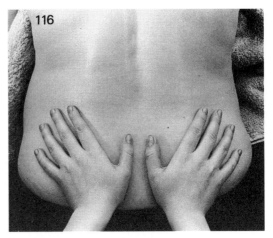

5) Lean thumbs into channels up either side of spine from sacrum to occiput, rotating the thumbs (fig. 114).

6) Knuckling along same lines either side of spine (fig. 115).

7) Effleurage over lumbar area 20 times (fig. 116).

8) Effleurage over upper back 20 times.

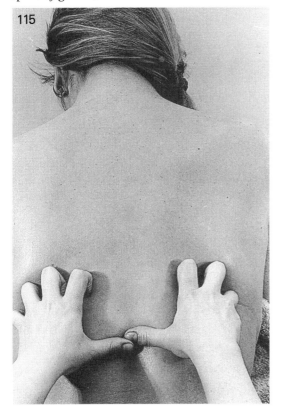

9) Rest one hand on one shoulder and lean other thumb into other side of back area between spine and shoulder blade. Work thumb around border of shoulder blade (fig. 117). Stand for this movement, swaying your weight into your thumb, bending the front legs.

10) Change hands and repeat on other side.

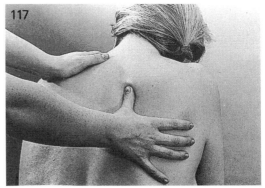

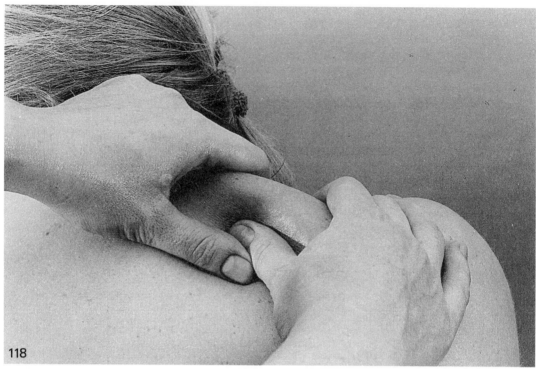

118

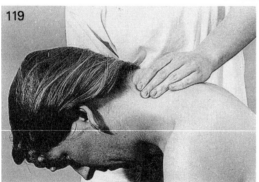

119

11) Squeeze and knead shoulder muscles one side at a time (*fig. 118*). Repeat on other side.

12) Stand to side of partner, cradling head in palm of one hand and lean other hand into neck and upwards to squeeze between fingers and thumbs (*fig. 119*). Change position to other side and repeat.

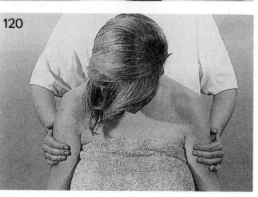

120

13) Stroke down the arms from the neck, over shoulders and down to hands (*fig. 120*). Squeeze both arms.

14) Effleurage once again from sacrum to back of skull at least ten times. Brush hands gently over forehead (*fig. 121*), head and down back to rest on lower back.

Note: It is possible to work on calves and feet in this position also.

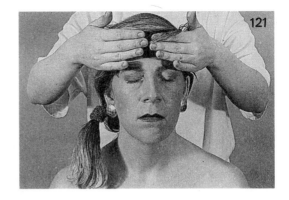

Side position Many of the strokes are the same as for the sitting sequence but are done one side at a time. Also, the giver's position is different, kneeling with the outside foot up, alongside the area to be massaged. You can also get further down the back in this position so it is useful to include the sacrum and buttocks (*figs. 122 and 123*). You can also reach over and give gentle abdominal massage with smooth strokes up over the abdomen to the side of the body (*fig. 124*).

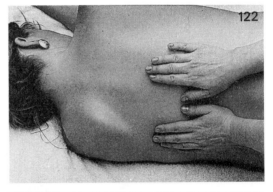

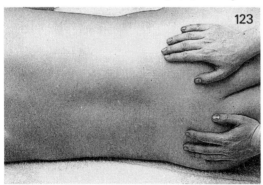

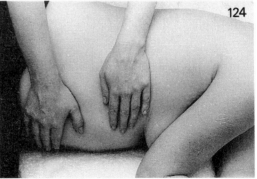

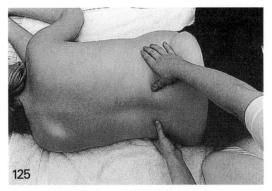

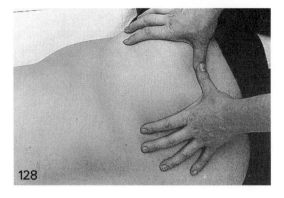

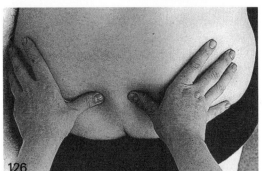

Points Concentrate on lower back and sacrum with a few shoulder points. UB 23 (fig. 125)— UB 34 (fig. 126), UB 52, 53, 54: for backache. GB 21 (fig. 127): for shoulder stiffness. Also GB 29, 30 (fig. 128) in side position: to increase circulation in legs and relieve tension in buttocks.

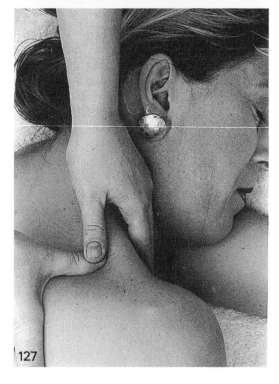

Abdomen This is the obvious place to massage during pregnancy and it is perfectly safe to do so provided soft, gentle pressure is used with no digging or kneading with the fingers. in the early stages it will help ease morning sickness, constipation and diarrhoea, whilst later on it will ease heartburn and indigestion as well as helping to prevent stretchmarks and ease taut skin. The baby itself will often respond to direct touch in this area and you may feel it move about, so this is a great way to communicate with the baby before it is born. In some cultures where midwives are well-trained in massage, such as India, abdominal massage may be used to change the position of a breech baby or generally encourage the baby to 'turn'. However, this may involve strong manipulation and is not advised here.

Sequence You may use the same basic sequence described in the menstruation chapter (*fig. 129*). The main things to remember are to give gentle, light pressure, flowing effleurage only. Even fingertip stroking can be effective (*fig. 130*). Cover the whole abdomen down to the groin and upper thigh. Remember, you are massaging two people now, so keep an image of the baby in your mind as you go. You can include breast massage here in the later stages of pregnancy to soften the breasts and nipples. Use almond oil as well.

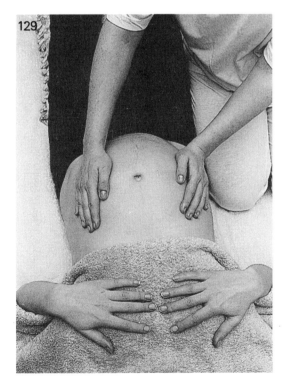

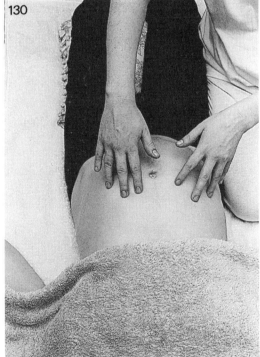

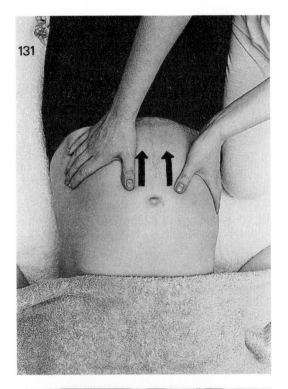

Points It is generally not a good idea to use pressure points directly on the abdomen during pregnancy. However, during effleurage, gentle thumb pressure along the meridians may be useful. Points along the stomach channel from 25 to 30 are good for relaxing the abdominal muscles, aiding digestion (*fig. 131*). Ki 11—16 (*fig. 132*) and CV 2—8 (*fig. 133*) will also affect the uterus and overall body energy, whilst CV 9—15 will help water retention, indigestion and heartburn.

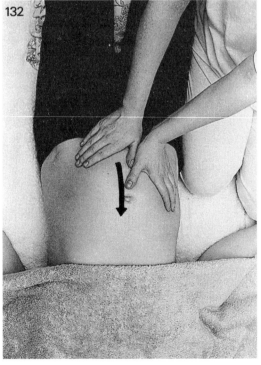

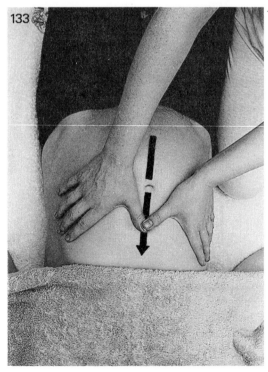

Legs and Feet

It is easy to massage the legs and feet whilst your partner is lying on her back, and this will enhance the effect of the abdominal massage. You can use finger pressure safely in this area with a wider variety of strokes including kneading and squeezing. The inner thigh is particularly responsive to pressure. Gently stretching the legs apart as you massage will help relax and tone the pelvic floor muscles which are crucial in the birth process. You may also reach the perineal area. It is vital to massage this area regularly because this will soften and stretch it, allowing for maximum aperture at birth and avoiding the risk of tearing. Regular massage to the legs will improve circulation and drainage and, especially in later pregnancy, help reduce the possibility of varicosities as well as muscle cramps.

Sequence Again, you may refer to the leg sequence described in the chapter on menstruation. One extra stroke you may try is to gently compress the palms together, one on each side of the thigh moving upward from the knee. Release, slide and press. Repeat on the other side. For the perineal massage as follows: (*fig. 133a*).

1) Receiver lies on back with legs apart. Use pillows under receiver's bottom to elevate the area. In early pregnancy she may equally lie on her front with pillows under her tummy.

2) Use fingertip pressure to massage the perineal area — between the vagina and the anus.

3) Use firm kneading pressure to the whole upper inside thigh right back as far as the tip of the sacrum. When lying on her front, buttock massage is also very effective.

Refer to Chapter 9 for foot massage but concentrate on the instep of the foot and the arch on the sole. These are areas which often get cramps.

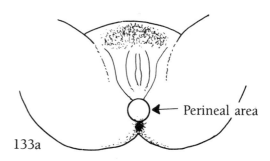

Perineal area

133a

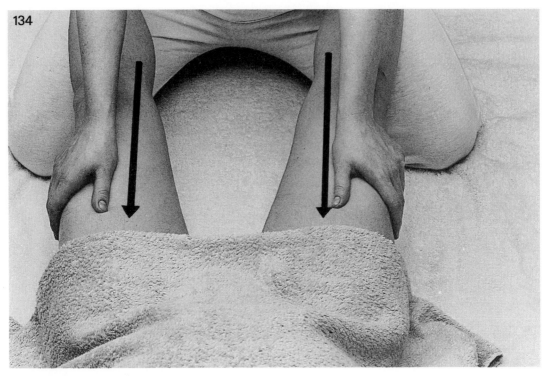

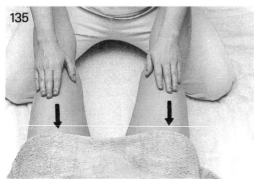

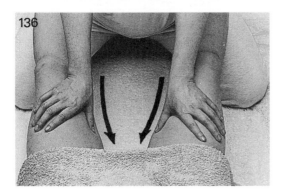

Points For thighs, follow the path of the spleen (*fig. 134*), liver (*fig. 135*) and kidney (*fig. 136*) meridians with your thumbs when doing effleurage. Important points in the perineal area are CV 1 and GV 1. For the lower legs, points along the inside of the legs are generally forbidden in pregnancy and you should avoid direct pressure on any spleen meridian points between Sp 6 and Sp 9, especially Sp 6 (*fig. 137*). Gentle stroking of these areas is OK. On the feet, points for cramps in the areas mentioned would include Ki 2 and Ki 1. (see page 68).

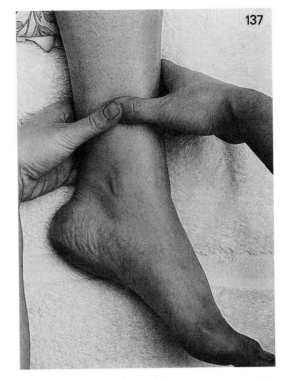

Miscellaneous points Pe 6 (*fig. 138*) has proved very effective in reducing the effects of morning sickness at the time it is experienced, though regular massage and shiatsu are a more effective preventative treatment. LI 4 (*fig. 139*) can be used for regulation of the bowel movement (constipation and diarrhoea) and for general well-being.

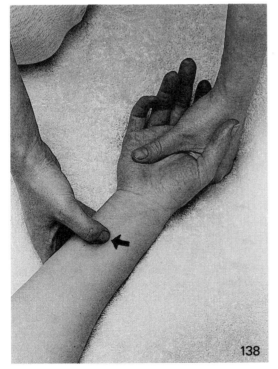

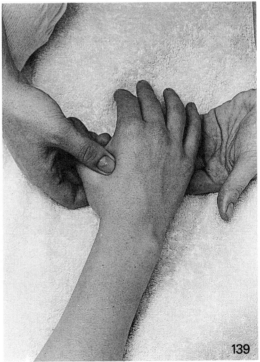

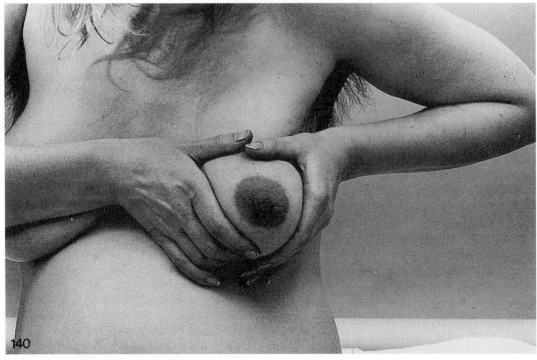

140

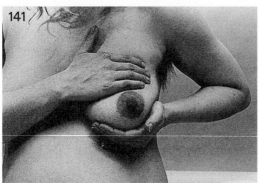

141

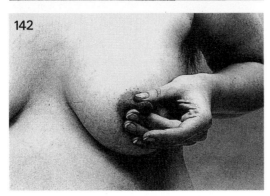

142

Self massage This can include most of the above but should include perineal massage and breast and nipple massage (good with almond oil) to soften and stretch these areas in preparation for birth and breastfeeding (*figs. 140, 141 and 142*).

Birth

There is no doubt that massage during the birth can be very beneficial to all concerned. It will help in regularizing contractions, relaxing muscles and easing pain and generally providing warmth and support for the mother and baby. If it is carried out by the father, it also allows him to take part in the birth experience. The main thing for him to remember is to be flexible! Your partner may not always want to be touched during labour, or she may just want fingertip pressure. You may have to shift your position regularly and adapt your strokes accordingly to what is happening or what your partner wants. It is easy to become tired or get in the way so endurance and patience may be needed. Often, it will be difficult to get at the torso, so massaging the face, neck, and shoulders, hands and feet are all possibilities. See relevant chapters for sequences. Where possible, back massage is very effective, especially on the sacrum from where all the nerves which run to the pelvis originate.

Points St 36 (*fig. 143*) will help regularize contractions and relieve pain. LI 4 will ease pain. Sp 6 will relax the uterus and speed delivery. UB 31 — 34 to ease back pain and speed delivery. UB 67 (*fig. 144*) is traditionally used to turn the baby when in breech but it may also aid a normal delivery. (For this point, use the edge of your fingernail and gently squeeze in at the corner of the toenail.)

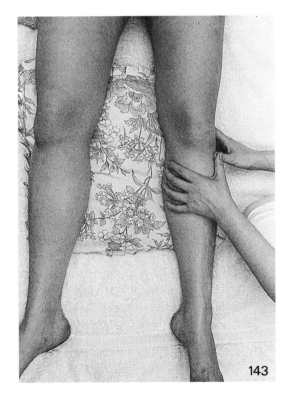

143

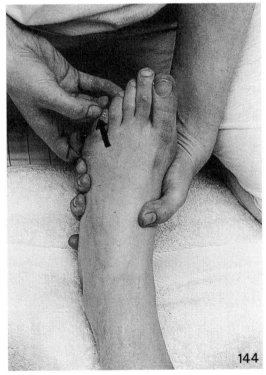

144

After birth

The period immediately following the birth and for up to a month afterwards is yet another time of great change for the woman. As a new mother, demands on her energy and time are great, yet she needs time to recover from the massive effort of carrying and giving birth to the baby. Her body needs to regenerate and readjust, yet it also needs training to get back into shape both internally and externally. The uterus as well as the pelvic and abdominal muscles must retract and contract and return to their normal shape and size. The lower back needs strengthening, the spine straightening and the neck and shoulders need relaxing after the tension caused by the weight of the baby. Finally, the mother will need good circulation and drainage to promote energy and vitality. Massage will help to achieve all these things.

In many cultures, postnatal care focuses greatly on the importance of massage. Many women in Africa are massaged daily following birth and their abdomens bound with cloth to prevent stretching. In China, the new mother is kept indoors, often lying down, for at least a month, though often massage or exercise will be prescribed. In some cases, the placenta is eaten and tonifying herbs taken for up to six months.

In any event, massage can help restore the mother both physically and emotionally following the birth. It can help deepen the couple's relationship and cement the bond between both parents and the baby (see next chapter). What could be a time of postpartum 'blues', where the mother may feel anti-social and tired, can be transformed through massage into a time of vibrant growth and development for the whole family. Intimate thoughts and experiences shared during this 'babymoon' time may positively affect the quality of relationship for all, later on.

Sequences It may only be possible to give a very gentle, fingertip stroking of the abdomen in the first few days following the birth. After a Caesarean, the scar area should obviously be avoided. However, neck and shoulder, back, leg and foot massages, as described earlier in this chapter, are all useful at this time. The main difference in massaging after birth as opposed to before is that, once you begin working on the abdomen, your pressure can be much firmer and can include kneading and squeezing techniques. Indeed these are essential for proper restoration of the abdominal muscles. Use the same points and meridians described earlier, although again, finger pressure directly on the points can be applied safely.

Self massage

This can be used in all the areas mentioned where possible but is mainly beneficial in two areas not always appropriately massaged by a partner: 1) The perineal area using fingertip pressure where there may be soreness or even slight tearing. Massage will speed the healing process. Use wheatgerm oil; use homoeopathic calendula tincture as well. Avoid the area if stitches are in place though gentle massage in the surrounding tissue, as with any other type of injury, can speed up recovery. 2) Breast massage will help the mother to express her milk, that is, to start the flow of milk without the baby's help. Cup the breast in your hands and use smooth, flowing effleurage from the periphery towards the centre and nipple until the milk comes. It is useful when the breasts are sore or overfull or when the mother wishes to keep a supply for later on. However, if the breasts are very painful as in mastitis, local massage will not help and the breasts will be too sore to touch. Massaging away from the breasts and chest area surrounding them may help move the congested blood and fluids. Any severe pain should be attended to by a physician.

Exercise

Prior to and after the birth it is essential for

the mother to take regular exercise. This may be general cardiovascular exercise simply to keep fit to deal with the excess demands being made on her system or it may be specific such as pelvic floor, abdominal and back exercise and breathing in preparation for the birth itself. In any event, the value of exercise during this crucial year or so of a woman's life is paramount — toning, firming and strengthening muscles, relaxing tension, increasing circulation, maintaining flexibility, reducing fatigue and revitalizing. Swimming is an obvious choice where the support of water, especially in the third trimester, makes exercise much more possible. Specific muscular exercise concentrating on pelvis, back and abdomen are too detailed to list here but there are many books available on the subject (see Bibliography). Join a yoga or active birth class.

Finally, regular and pre- and postnatal exercise will undoubtedly reduce the risk of long-term ill-effects of childbirth such as prolapse of the uterus, varicose veins and haemorrhoids.

7

Babies and infants

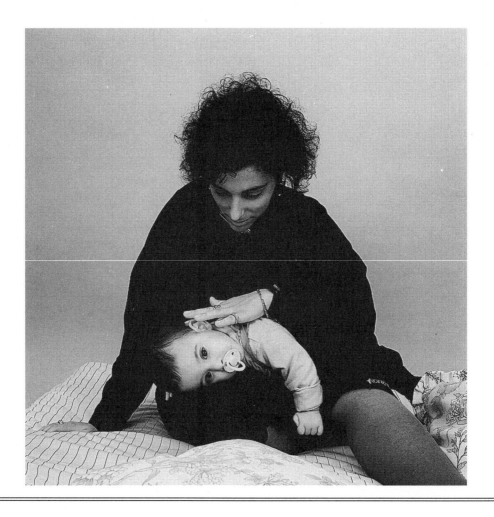

The Jesuit adage 'Give me a child before the age of seven and he is mine for life' points to the vital period of infancy and early childhood in the forming of the individual. By the age of seven a child has developed functionally and behaviourally to a degree that may predetermine the rest of his or her experience of life. We have already discussed the role of touch in the physiological development of the newborn, its influence on body systems, especially the nervous system, and its role in influencing, if not determining, behavioural patterns in later life. A few salient points on the role of massage and loving touch in the early years of life may serve to highlight the case even further.

Babies enjoy their first experience of touch and massage when they are still in the womb, being constantly caressed by the warm amniotic fluid they have been encased in. Touch is the first sense that they develop (in the womb). Then as the baby moves from this home to the outside world, s/he is gently squeezed and pushed by the strong muscles in the birth canal. By the time the baby enters the world s/he is already familiar with touch as reassuring and comforting.

Active birth

Attitudes towards the birth process and the role of touch have dramatically changed in recent years. The Active Birth movement started by Janet Balaskas is a reflection of our desire to get back in touch with the whole process of birth and involve ourselves and our partners more actively in it. It emphasizes the importance of making the baby's potentially traumatic transition from the warm, safe environment of the womb as smooth and easy as possible.

Soothing music, soft lighting, active, responsive 'helpers' and even water all help in this transition. Gentle rocking by the mother as soon as the baby is born even helps recreate the position, warmth and gentle movement of the amniotic fluid it has just left. The common factor in both environments is touch, whether direct tactile stimulation, or temperature which is also sensed by the skin. Babies are ultra-sensitive to touch and to temperatures, responding positively to the quality of soft, soothing touch and to heat. Both of course are provided by the mother, most obviously in the first year of life by rocking, caressing, and breastfeeding. Certain areas of the skin, such as the hands, especially the thumb and forefinger, and the lips, are extremely highly sensitized. Is it any wonder then that a baby's first impressions of the world around it are gathered through messages received by fingering and sucking things?

Perhaps less obvious is the fact that babies are highly sensitive to the gestures and movements of the people they are in contact with. They can tell for example what state of mind their mother is in by sensing her muscular reactions and vibrations, a process known as kinaesthetic sensation.

The role of the father in the early days and weeks of infancy is important. It can be an invaluable time to create a relationship with the baby, and establish an active parenting role. The new father can easily learn to massage his new baby and spend quality time with him/her. It gives him a wonderful way to soothe and calm his child.

This can also benefit the mother greatly: she may easily feel overwhelmed at the enormity of her responsibilities. The father's close involvement at this time also handles any feelings of exclusion he may encounter.

The baby's new world appears very different from the old one. Depending on the particular environment they are born into, the world can seem cold, harsh and unappealing or warm and supportive. We can do much to ease this transition by giving birth in a peaceful, softly-lit room with soothing music and gentle lights. However, giving babies constant, loving and reassuring touch is a much-neglected way of adding a familiar sensation to their new world. Touch, above all the other senses, is the first and most important to develop after birth. It is through touch that the new baby experiences the new environment and relationship with other humans. They will learn how valued, how loved, how welcome and how important they are through the quality of touch we extend to them. Above all they will experience their new world as a safe, welcoming place to be: and other people as loving, supportive and safe to be with. We have to remember that the baby was in a very safe, warm and comfortable place where all their needs were met and their move to a strange environment may have felt like a painful, forceful ejection.

In such a world, completely dominated by the sense of touch, massage can be used to great advantage. As well as assisting in the natural physiological development of the baby, it will contribute to well-balanced, integrated behaviour which reduces the chance of psychological or emotional problems later in life. Naturally, it helps create a close, loving bond between mother or father and child. This is a crucial contribution to what can be a very trying time for any relationship. Massaging the baby as well as massaging one another is a great way to ease tensions and contribute to one another. Later on, the child can learn to give massage too.

Bonding

The very early days of its new life are when the baby will form its primary conclusions and decisions about this new world, and people. It is no overstatement to say that the quality of touch we can offer new babies sets them up for life to feel safe and secure with other human beings. Babies who are born through Caesarean section, premature or incubated and who miss out on the massage through the birth canal, need even more amounts of touch and massage. They also miss out on the bonding with the mother, and may find close-

ness and intimacy with other people difficult, even from the early days onwards! It is reputed that a high proportion of present-day computer geniuses began life in an incubator, so their first intimate, bonding life-saving relationship was with a machine! Massage for the Caesarean baby offers the possibility of feeling safe and loved with another human being.

For the fast-birth baby, massage is also important, but for different reasons. The baby who, due to the speed of their birth, misses out on the birth canal massage, misses out on the sensation and experience of feeling the separateness and entirety of their physical body, unlike being in the womb where there was no distinction between their own body and the womb.

It is believed that fast-birth babies might later feel ambiguous about their body and be overly head-oriented people. They would benefit enormously from massage which would bring them back into their bodies and encourage them to feel acceptance towards their bodies. Children who receive trust and confidence through the early touch of their parents are much more likely to express confidence, security and independence as individuals from very early on in their lives.

Observation has shown that babies and children who are deprived of touch generally suffer from anxiety and its related disorders. In fact babies can actually waste away and die from a disease called marasmus if they do not receive enough loving touch. Following the Second World War studies were undertaken to discover the cause of marasmus. It was found to occur most frequently in affluent homes and hospitals and least among poor households. What was less obvious in the first group and abundant in the second was tender loving care.

Several American hospitals recognized this in the late 1920s and consequently introduced systematic mothering where babies were picked up and cuddled and carried around several times a day. In one hospital, Bellvue Hospital in New York, following the introduction of 'mothering', the mortality rates for infants under one year fell from 30—35 per cent to less than 10 per cent within a few years.

The baby, therefore, needs to be handled and caressed frequently, in order to thrive. This is common among the cultures of Africa, the Caribbean and India where the baby is 'stretched' immediately after birth following the physical confinement in the womb. Massage promotes flexibility and suppleness in the muscles and joints and helps prepare the baby to co-ordinate its body. This is particularly true when the baby is getting ready to walk.

Acclimatization

The specific value of massage to babies and infants is firstly to acclimatize them to their own bodies — a new distraction for them as they learn to cope with the sudden impact of previously unknown forces upon them, namely, air and gravity. The first great shock to the baby's system is the sudden inflation of the lungs — its first breath. Next comes the need to nourish itself, since its automatic food supply, the umbilical cord, has been cut. Once these basic needs have met, the baby can begin to investigate its new world, and the first years of its life are concerned with learning to master its own body movements and functions.

Massage can play a part in assisting the baby through all these vital stages. It affects the respiratory system by relaxing and toning all the muscles involved in the breathing process, and by calming the nervous system, promoting deeper, slower more rhythmic breaths. Through kinaesthetic sensing, the baby may also learn to 'tune into' and follow the mother's breathing pattern and rhythm. This is also true of the heartbeat and rhythm. The effects of massage in aiding digestion are well-known. It improves absorption and elimination. Interestingly, many early childhood illnesses are concerned with respiratory, digestive and muscular dysfunctions, whether voluntary or involuntary. Crying, coughs, nasal congestions, asthma, stomach ache, indigestion, wind, vomiting, poor appetite, constipation and diarrhoea, tiredness, listlesness, bedwetting — all such complaints are associated with one or more of the above functions.

Oriental medicine offers a useful parallel to this chronology of physiological development within the newborn baby. It draws attention the natural cycle of Ki or Chi — the vital life force motivating all things. According to them it has a clear cycle of activity throughout the body, passing from one organ system to another, conducted along the meridians, beginning with the lung and ending with the liver.

It is not sufficiently clear from the classics, or at least it has not been made clear by teachers of the subject, why the cycle should begin with the lung. Yet the tissue associated with the lungs in ancient medicine is the skin, the orifice it controls is the nose, and it is said to control exchanges and transmissions with the environment. This concurs exactly with the function of the *ectoderm*, the outer layer of the growing embryo, later to become the skin, which provides the organism with information about the environment. The *mesoderm*, the middle layer of the developing embryo, later develops into the muscles. Here again there is an interesting connection in oriental medicine.

The second organ in the cycle of energy flow is the system which controls transformation and transportation of nutrients. The tissue associated with it is the muscles and the orifice it controls is the mouth. Along with their associated 'hollow' organs — lung with large intestine; spleen with stomach — they account for the two primary life functions in early life — breathing and eating.

If we expand these functions to include the related organs in Chinese medicine, the skin and muscles, the nose and the mouth, we have a comprehensive picture of the natural way a baby instinctively seems to stimulate these functions. When breastfeeding, massive tactile stimulation of the nose and mouth occur, whilst the baby continually seeks to be touched and handled. Massage is obviously a way of maintaining and increasing the amount of overall touch the baby will receive, and the implication is that it assists in the healthy development of respiratory and digestive function.

It would be interesting to find out for example the relationship between later-life disorders of these systems, especially nervous-related ones such as asthma, skin allergies, hiatus hernia, ulcers and colitis, and the relative amount of touch and massage received during early childhood.

Massage and Shiatsu

We have seen how massage, from birth through infancy and childhood, can affect healthy development of the internal organs, the muscles and behaviour patterns. It will contribute towards a strong, healthy body, normal motor development and a calm, relaxed mentality. The main thing to remember in working on babies and young children is to be responsive to their moods and physical and mental condition. They easily get tired and their attention span is very short. It is important not to try to massage them when they are overtired, hungry or have just eaten or when something else is preoccupying them such as food, a game or a person. A warm environment and warm, manicured hands are important. Above all, a firm light-hearted approach, integrated with game-playing, tickling and stroking is more effective than a serious series of 'techniques'. Massage should be short and integrated into the day at obvious moments such as when not feeding, bathing or doing domestic work. It is important for the massage time to be a welcome relief from daily duties and it should be enjoyable for both parties. It will cease to be helpful if it becomes a 'chore'. Finally, hand pressure must be very light and gentle — light stroking is enough.

Shiatsu

In China, acupuncturists don't always insert the needle into the skin when treating babies. Instead they use a variety of instruments, mostly blunt, to tap, scrape and generally stimulate the surface of the skin. This is an indication of the extreme sensitivity of the skin as well as the baby's ability to recover quickly from minor ailments. Similarly with shiatsu, pressure need only be very gentle and light brushing of the meridians is perfectly effective, no need to press strongly into points. Gentle stretching is also very effective. Because babies are so flexible, it is quite easy and safe to perform. General body shiatsu is very effective for calming the baby and treating nervous disorders such as temper tantrums, hyperactivity, and bedwetting. Here are some areas to concentrate on.

Arms, chest and face
Shiatsu in these areas can principally affect the functioning of the lungs and large intestines which may help in a variety of respiratory ailments including coughs, sore throats, nasal and chest congestion and asthma.

1) Baby lies on its back.

2) Gentle thumb pressure and stroking along the lung and large intestine meridians holding the hand in one hand and giving sliding pressure with the other (fig. 144a). Concentrate on Lu 10 when there is a sore inflamed throat and on Lu 6 when coughing or asthma is acute. Concentrate on LI 11 for allergies such as infantile eczema; LI 4 for constipation as well as head and nasal congestion.

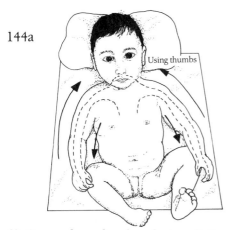

144a

from extra point Yintang to GV 23. UB 2 is very effective for clearing a stuffy head.

Abdomen and legs

Digestive disorders are also very common in babies and infants and can be much relieved by shiatsu to the legs and abdomen, mainly along the stomach and spleen meridians. Use the following sequences to treat tummy upsets, indigestion and wind as well as constipation, diarrhoea and urogenital problems.

1) Baby lies on back.

2) Gentle stroking pressure along stomach and spleen meridians starting in groin area and moving up torso to neck. Emphasize St 25 for constipation and diarrhoea as well as stomach upsets and wind (fig. 144c).

3) Come above head and give sliding pressure in between first, second and third ribs from the sternum in the centre out to the side of the body (fig. 144b). These points may be sore so be gentle. Points to remember Lu 1/2, good for coughs and asthma.

4) Thumb sliding pressure along side and front of neck for soothing coughs and relieving sore throats (fig. 144b).

5) On the face, use the same basic sequence described in Chapter 9 but adapt the pressure and intensity to the baby. Concentrate on LI 20 for nasal congestion as well as points up the side of the nose and on the midline

3) Give sliding pressure along conception vessel from the pelvic bone up to the ribcage. Emphasize CV 10/12 and 13 for digestive and elimination problems, (fig. 144d) and CV 3/4 and 6 for bedwetting.

Note: For a complete abdominal treatment of digestive problems give clockwise circular palm pressure over the umbilicus and then gradually outwards to include CV 12, CV4, and Sp 15 at each extremity (fig. 144d).

144b

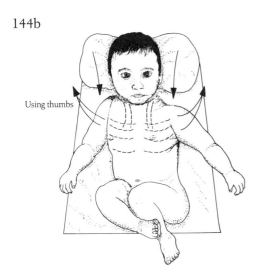

144c

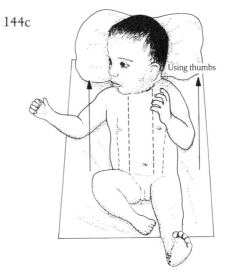

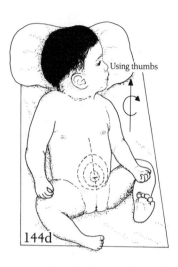

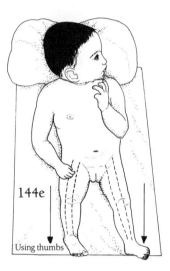

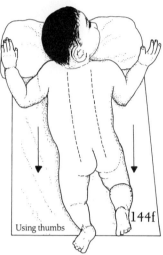

4) Move the legs and give thumb sliding pressure down the legs both on the inside and outside near the bone following the stomach and spleen meridians (*fig. 144e*). Emphasize St 36/37 and 39 as well as Sp 6.

Back

The points along the bladder meridian on the back have direct associations with all the internal organs and can thus be used to regulate many digestive and respiratory problems when used in conjunction with the above sequences (*fig. 144f*).

1) Sliding thumb pressure on the upper back alongside spine as far as UB 15. These points will often help coughs and asthma as well as anxiety and irritability.

2) Sliding thumb pressure on the mid-back alongside spine from UB 20. These points will help most digestive disorders.

3) Same techniques as the lower back and sacrum from UB 23 to 34 emphasizing UB 23, 31, 32, 33 and 34 for bedwetting and UB 25 for constipation.

Exercise

Naturally, young babies and infants exercise themselves through learning to move around, first on their bottoms, then all fours and finally walking. To increase the speed of this development and to help co-ordination and balance, gentle stretching is useful to compliment the baby's own movements.

Child sits on the floor with legs out in front of them. Kneel behind them and allow your knee to support their back. Bring the hands over their head holding at wrists. Lean back, holding knee in place, and stretch whole body back. This movement especially stretches the abdomen, legs and inside of the arms and affects the stomach, spleen and lung meridians whose significance we have discussed.

Finally, it should be mentioned that massage and shiatsu are generally contraindicated when the baby or infant is suffering from chills or fevers, though moxa can be used.

Bach flower remedies

Bach flower remedies can be safely given to babies of three months and upwards. They should be diluted: one drop to a small cup of warm water. Prior to three months, the remedy bottle can simply be placed beside the baby and the particular vibration from the remedy will be sufficient to make a difference. Though your baby cannot speak directly to you of their mental or emotional turmoil they may express it through physical symptoms and it will be up to you to discern what the underlying trouble might be:

The birth experience, guilt following a traumatic birth, the baby may feel to blame for the pain caused to the mother:
Pine

Shock, following a forceps or induced birth, the baby may be experiencing acute shock — or the umbilical cord was cut very soon after the baby had taken its first breath:
Star of Bethlehem

Resentment, bitterness — appropriate if the baby has had to be induced or brought out with forceps:
Willow

Fearfulness — following forceps or induced birth:
Rock rose

Anxiety — if baby had cord around neck:
Cherry, plum

Later on the baby may benefit from the following:

Getting used to new surroundings — use in first days of their arrival:
Walnut

Impatience, irritability:
Impatiens

Anxiety for no known reason:
Aspen

Rescue Remedy can also be used at times of great distress or emergency.

Oils

Oils can be of great benefit to babies and can be used, with care, when children are a few weeks old. Obviously the dilution of essential oil to vegetable oil is much greater than for adults: for every two tablespoons of vegetable oil use three drops of essential oils. Never use the oils undiluted in baby's bath as you would do for yourself. This is because the oils will stay on the surface of the water and the baby may well rub some into its eyes. The oils can be added to two tablespoons of oil or to a cup of creamy milk and mixed well before adding to the bath. Your baby's delicate skin will benefit greatly from using almond oil because it is very nourishing without being heavy.

Commercial baby oil should not be used. It is a mineral oil and does not absorb into the skin.

Stomach upsets/colic/digestive
Camomile and Lavender are very soothing oils and are best used here in massage directly on the tummy. Of the three types of Camomile available, Camomile Romain is the best for a baby's skin because it is non-toxic.

Teething
Camomile and Lavender: massage gently into the cheeks. Use Camomile first but if the baby prefers the aroma of Lavender this will also will be effective.

Sleeplessness
Lavender — Use in night time baths, massage. Inhalation — place a drop on the baby's pillow.

Skin irritation/nappy rash
Camomile — Use in massage, in baths. Calendula cream is also recommended for nappy rash.

Coughs/colds/respiratory problems
Eucalyptus; Benzoin; Frankincense; Myrrh. Eucalyptus is effective in the treatment of a cough or cold. This can be massaged into the baby's chest and back and drops placed on their pillow to help during sleep. Benzoin is similarly effective and can be used in the same way. Frankincense is particularly beneficial for breathing difficulties. Use in massage and on the baby's pillow. Myrrh is excellent for soothing inflammation of the bronchial tubes and expelling mucus. Use in massage and on the baby's pillow.

Self-esteem

The time from birth to five years is now widely acknowledged as the most formative in determining the individual's sense of self and identity. Infants are extremely receptive to their parents' thoughts and attitudes towards them and may well reflect these in later life. Therefore it is very important to hold the highest quality thoughts you can towards children.

Baby massage — sequences

Massaging your baby is extremely simple and immensely rewarding for both baby and giver. There are no special strokes or techniques: it is just a matter of adapting the strokes and your hands to a tiny baby. Babies will feel the cold much more quickly than adults so the room will have to be extremely warm. Keep a spare blanket and towel by you. Because the baby will be naked, place a towel underneath in case of accidents. Use an oil like almond or coconut but not baby oil as it is a mineral oil and not beneficial to the skin. The following sequences are a guideline for you and you will want to extend your repertoire by inventing your own strokes. Begin massaging your baby immediately, being attentive to their response and avoid the navel area until it has healed. It's very pleasant to lay the baby on your legs as you do the massage so they get as much skin contact as possible.

Face

It's good to begin on the face so you can have eye contact with your baby as they get used to your strokes. Lay the baby on your knees, with their feet pointing up and have your back well supported. Talk gently to your baby throughout the massage.

1) Stroke your baby's forehead from the centre outwards to the hairline, with your thumbs. Keep the rest of your hands relaxed and in contact with the face (fig. 145). Repeat.

2) Stroke across the cheeks from the nose outwards with the thumbs. Hands in contact with rest of face (fig. 146). Repeat.

3) Place your thumbs above the upper lip and stroke up to the ear (fig. 147). Repeat.

4) Squeeze jawline gently between fingers and thumbs from the centre out to each ear. Repeat (fig. 148).

5) Squeeze ears gently (fig. 149).

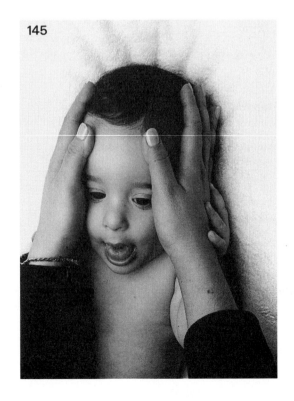

145

146

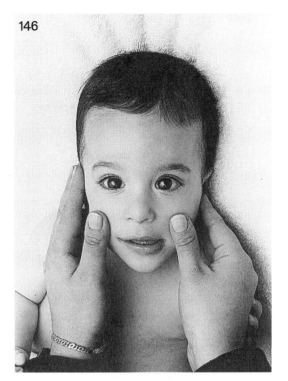

147

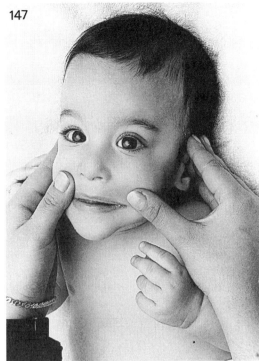

148

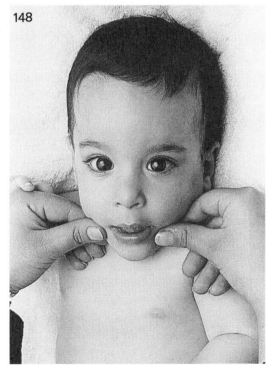

149

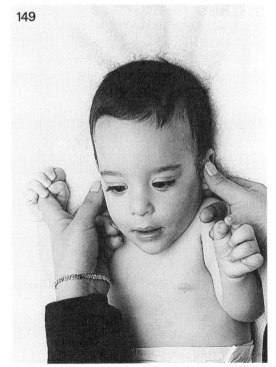

Chest

1) Glide oil over whole front of body, chest and abdomen, arms and legs.

2) Rest hands on upper chest and spread out towards each arm stroking down sides of torso and sweep back onto chest (*fig. 150*). Repeat.

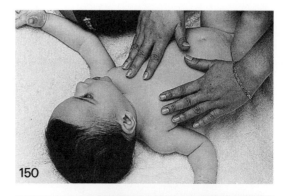

3) Circle flat fingers over chest, sides of torso and back onto chest (*fig. 151*). Repeat.

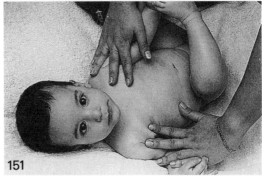

Abdomen

1) Rest hands on abdomen and circle slowly around the navel in a clockwise direction. Lift right hand over the left as they cross (*fig. 152*). This movement is useful for colic and digestive upsets.

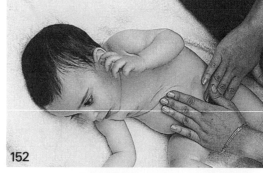

2) Stroke up the abdomen, chest, out over the shoulders and down the arms (*fig. 153*). Sweep back onto the abdomen and stroke down abdomen and over legs.

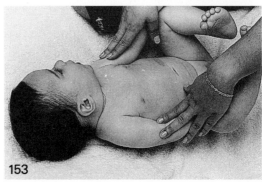

Arms

1) Hold baby's hand and stroke down their arm from the shoulder with other hand (*fig. 154*). Repeat.

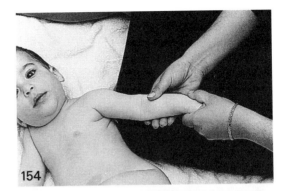

2) Squeeze the arm gently from the shoulder downwards (*fig. 155*). Repeat.

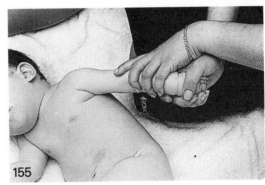

3) Slide thumbs over back of hand. Hold hand at wrist and with your other hand squeeze each finger between your finger and thumb (*fig. 156*).

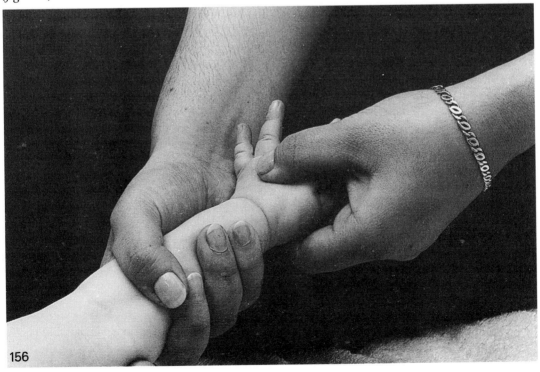

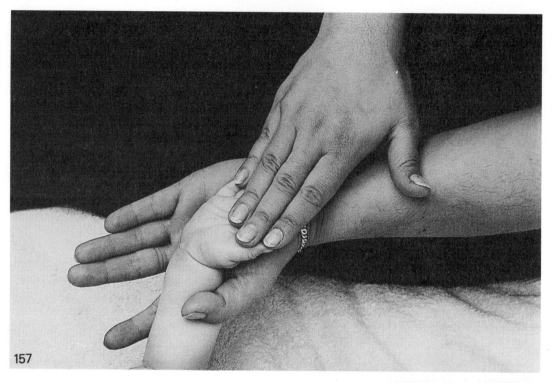

157

4) Turn the hand over and hold at wrist. Spread your other hand over their palm, uncurling the fingers as you glide your hand over them (*fig. 157*). Repeat. Repeat this sequence on other arm.

Legs
1) Hold the foot in one hand and stroke down the leg from thigh to foot (*fig. 158*). Repeat.

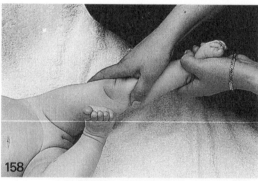

158

2) Squeeze the leg from thigh to foot (*fig. 159*). Repeat.

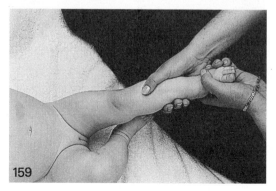

159

3) Stretch up leg. Hold ankle and glide your hand over the sole of the foot (*fig. 160*). Squeeze each toe between finger and thumb (*fig. 161*). Repeat this sequence on other leg.

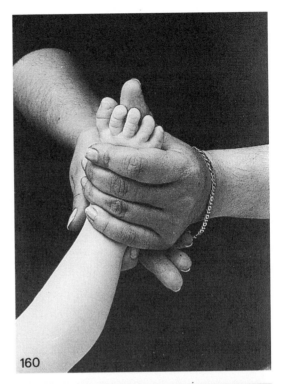

160

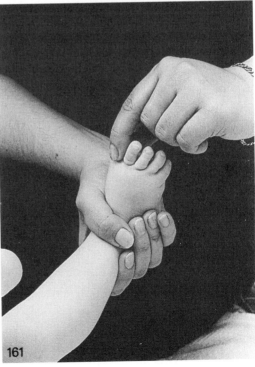

161

Back

Turn your baby over and lay it across your legs on its tummy.

1) Glide oil over back and legs starting at the top of the back (*fig. 162*).

2) Wring your hand back and forth across the back and buttocks (*fig. 163*).

3) Glide thumbs up the back along either side of spine (*fig. 164*).

4) Stroke buttocks and squeeze gently (*fig. 165*).

5) Complete by stroking one hand after the other down the back and over the legs (*fig. 166*).

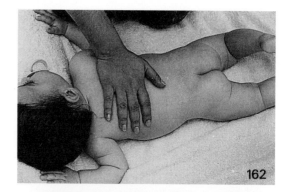

162

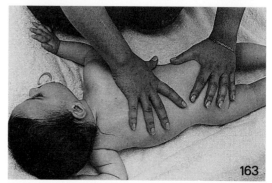

163

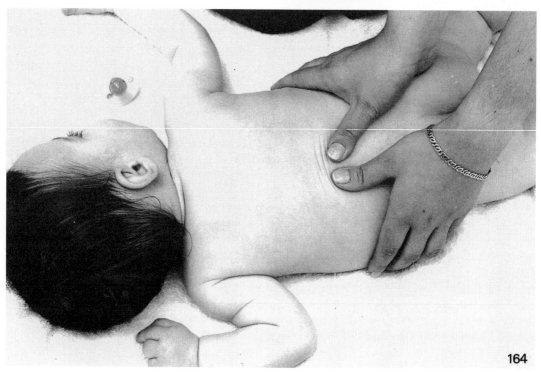

164

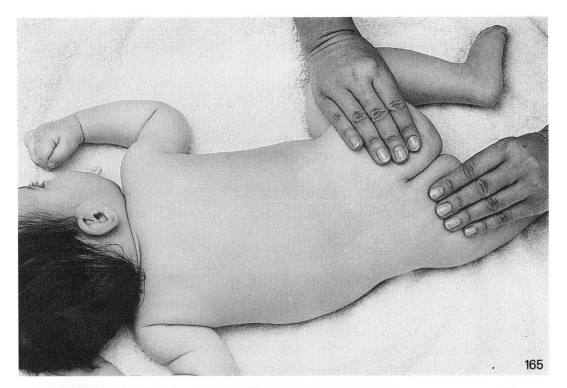

165

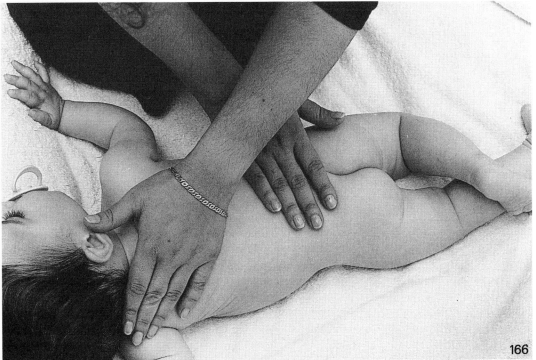

166

8

Adolescence

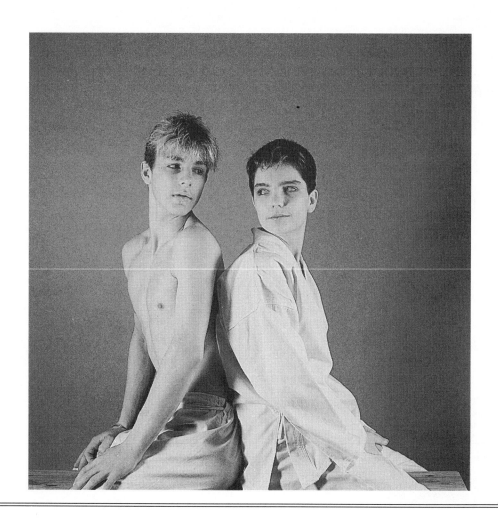

The onset of puberty and adolescence brings with it a whole series of major changes for the young person. Not least of these is the abrupt cessation of touch and skin contact. As a child they would have enjoyed immense amounts of cuddling and embracing, maybe including sleeping with parents. But at the age of about 13, a lot of parental contact becomes taboo and the young person begins to guard her/his developing body and sexuality.

At the same time they are also beginning to experience much greater skin sensitivity and the young adolescent discovers the sensitivity of touch as never before. The adolescent child is growing into a world of sexuality where touch may stimulate thoughts and desires they feel uncomfortable with. As a result of this new sensuality, young people draw away from the reassurance of touch they previously enjoyed. It is during this time and the forthcoming years that they need loving touch more than ever to feel safe and supported. At no other time in their forthcoming lives are they likely to feel more unsure of themselves or so overwhelmed by the hormonal changes in their bodies. At no other time are they likely to have less physical contact as they withdraw from parental touch and other physical relationships are prohibited.

It is little wonder then that adolescence is such a difficult and fraught time and that young people have increasingly resorted to alcohol and a variety of drugs and suppressants to 'get out of their heads' and become 'mindless'. Skin starvation may well have a large part to play in creating the need for reality-altering substances. Research carried out during the 1950s showed that monkeys deprived of touch grew up to be violent and delinquent.

When we are lacking in caring human touch, we are having our most basic primitive need denied us. Such a huge need that is never fulfilled inevitably leads to the young person feeling unloved, and very alone and cut off. They feel isolated and remote from everyone, including their peers, seeking approval and acceptance through any means. Seeking approval and acceptance can take on many forms, not all destructive. It may be cha..nelled into academic excellence or sporting prowess but very often can lead to competition with alcohol or drugs. Eating disorders such as anorexia nervosa and bulimia are extremely common among adolescent girls and are surely an expression of profound insecurity and uncertainty. Both disorders may also be an attempt to deny the physical changes taking place and to establish control over their bodies at a time when everything else in their lives is beyond their control.

No longer 'in touch'

Adolescents frequently complain that they have no say over their lives and decisions are made for them without taking them into consideration. This is often the case and reflects a poor relationship between parents and the new young adult: and this in turn reflects the physical situation that parents and their child are no longer in touch.

Many of the difficulties and traumas associated with this stage of life could be dealt with very easily if the young person could enjoy the deep feeling of being loved and cared for that s/he has grown accustomed to. The famous 'generation gap' between teenager and adults could be a thing of the past: and the young adult would be less needy for skin contact and less likely to crave sexual relations. It is at this time that adolescents learn to associate touch with sex: which is understandable if the only physical contact they can find is through sex. Teenage problems and poor relationships with adults could be transformed if the new adult could feel loved and appreciated. The only profound way they will feel this is through the physical contact they have grown up with, and which all human beings need. We cannot lead happy, contented lives without it, and we cannot survive without it.

The teenage years invariably make a strong and lasting impression on all of us. Whether we remember them fondly or otherwise, experiences we have and decisions we make at that time can often substantially affect the rest of our lives. We reach puberty, a bewildering and often upsetting period of intense physical and emotional change. Having spent most of the early years growing and adapting with the support of parents, identifying with them, and depending on them, we are suddenly faced with a new reality. We experience our bodies and ourselves for the first time as our gender claims and identifies us. This often brings up feelings of independence, even rebellion. The search to establish our own individual identity begins.

Social pressures

Yet mixed with this intensely personal process of physical and metaphysical transformation are some of the most severe and dogmatic social pressures we ever have to face. Although the gender divide is less obvious that it used to be, boys are still more likely to be faced with the dreaded 'and what are you going to be when you grow up?', while girls may be asked 'and who are you going to marry?' Although innocent enough in themselves, these simple demands made early in an adolescent's life can begin to give them the impression that their parents and relatives are trying to pressure them into submission. Some young men cannot help but emulate their fathers, while others try their utmost not to be like them. Daughters likewise with their mothers. Career and marriage pressures begun in mid to late teens can cause trauma for some adolescents at the very time they are struggling with finding their own identity. It then becomes easy for parents, role models for their offspring until that point, to suddenly become 'the enemy'.

Teenagers often turn to their peers at this time for support. While they may find like minds to identify with, peers do not always provide a very balanced view of the whole process and may often indulge a young person's less disciplined tendencies. Experiments with new-found sexual identity at this time are also based on the same desire to be different and to establish an identity. This can lead to the distorted importance of sexual gratification without a substantial relationship to back it up.

Adolescence is associated with a time of stifling responsibility. Familiar feelings amongst young people are loneliness, isolation and confusion. A common reaction is often frustration, anger and the desire to find a scapegoat. The psychlogical reasons behind many behavioural problems associated with adolescence can be complex and involve particular traumas like parental divorce, physical and sexual abuse, illness or extreme poverty. It is perhaps not surprising that such problems as bullying, vandalism and sexual violence, as well as self-abuse through such things as alcohol and drugs and over- or undereating (bulimia and anorexia) are usually begun during this period of one's life.

It is a time when we begin systematically to lose touch with one another, literally. Our parents no longer afford us the wealth of love through touch that they did, especially more recently with the scare of the 'sexual abuse' label. Fathers particularly have radically reduced their level of physical contact with their daughters for fear of such normal parental affection being misinterpreted. For their part teenagers, struggling with their new-found physical and sexual identity, steer away from overt parental affection. This is especially apparent among boys. Instead, they are condemned to the bravado of peer contact — a brusque slap on the back, a handshake. Close, full body contact becomes a thing of the past, indeed is actively avoided where possible. How the young teenager hates it when the mother says 'go on dear, give your auntie a kiss!'

It could be argued that the potentially traumatic experience of adolescence affects boys even more than girls and may account for the relatively poor quality of touch behaviour in men as opposed to women in later life. The young infant tends strongly and quite naturally to identify with his or her mother. This bond is generally accepted to be stronger than with the father. In early adolescence, as the child gradually establishes its own distinct identity, it is clear that such a process is potentially more traumatic for the boy than for the girl. In becoming a woman, the young girl has many adjustments to make. Yet all are within the context of womanhood. The mother does not appear as a threat in this respect, at least not immediately! For the boy however, as well as the physical and emotional upheaval of puberty, he must necessarily cease to identify with his role model — a woman — and assume his own identity as a man. Yet the closest person for him to identify with at this time, his father, may appear as almost a complete stranger to him. This must surely foster and exacerbate already developing feelings of identity crisis and alienation.

Massage and Shiatsu

Massage, when fully and naturally incorporated into family life from an early age, can help bridge this potential gap between parent and child. It can give each a legitimate opportunity to be intimate and to help develop a more comprehensive definition of touch, not just associated with sex. It gives time to the young person, and to the parent, to just 'be', to relax and allow someone else to support them, to 'let them in', or more accurately 'let them back in'. Above all, massage will help restore self-esteem in the growing adolescent, fraught with fears and fixations about physical appearance, about mannerisms and about whether they are liked or disliked. It is perhaps the greatest and simplest gift imaginable to them, saying clearly and without innuendo 'I love and care for you'. For the parents too, it is an invaluable way

to lessen the experience of 'losing' their babies.

It is difficult to ascribe a specialist role to any form of hands-on therapy during adolescence. For the most part, it is a time when general health is flourishing, the body is defining itself and getting stronger every day. The only common minor physical ailments associated with this stage of life tend to be limited to the hormonal change brought on by puberty. In boys in particular this can lead to acne and other skin conditions. However, as we have already identified, the emotional change of this period can cause major behavioural problems in young adults. The effect of any kind of touch then, given the right approach and environments, will help stabilize hormonal imbalance, reduce stress and tension and encourage a calmer, more rational appreciation of this temporary 'phase' of life.

Massage increases the flexibility and elasticity of the skin and encourages it to 'breathe' more efficiently. It also helps balance hormone secretion and regulation, especially of androgen, the sex hormone that controls the secretion of sebum. An excess of it can cause acne. Massage will help the sebaceous glands (the obstruction of which can also cause acne) to function healthily. it will also aid circulation of blood and lymph to nourish and cleanse the body.

Many adolescents, particularly boys, will not always welcome the idea of being massaged. This will be especially true of those who did not receive regular touch or massage when they were younger. So parents or peers must find ways in which structured touching will be acceptable to young adults. One way is to remind them of the importance of developing a strong and healthy body. For boys, this may involve reminding them that athletes and sports people often receive regular massage to stay fit. Naturally, as discussed in Chapter 10, this is in fact totally legitimate. Massage during this period of massive physical development is an ideal way to encourage muscle and bone growth, flexibility and strength. It is also a way to encourage good posture and avoid the possibility of poor holding patterns that develop through tension and imbalance. For girls, who tend to have less of 'touch taboo', it may be useful to highlight the important of massage in helping balance hormone secretion and distribution. See Chapter 5 for details on how massage can be used to help problems associated with the onset of puberty.

Naturally, at a time when adolescents are discovering their sexuality, touch is often easily interpreted in a sensual way and the approach and practice of it needs careful thought and management. It is as perfect a time as any to share the benefits of increased intimacy in a perfectly natural, open way to try to counter some of the acute loneliness and isolation sometimes experienced by adolescents in this phase of their lives.

Shiatsu

The meridians most closely associated with emotional upheaval caused by hormonal imbalance are the liver and kidney meridians. (We have seen that where menstruation is concerned this includes the spleen — see Chapter 5.) Where psychological disturbances occur such as panic attacks and anxiety and worry with symptoms like insomnia and palpitations, the heart and pericardium meridians may also be invovled. We have discussed the relationships in Oriental medicine between the lung and the skin as a symbol of the relationship between the self and the environment, so any crisis of identity and communication or relationship problems may involve the lung meridians.

So, it is clear that such a period involves changes which affect the workings of the entire body. Symptomatic massage, unless it is a quick five-minute rub down for neck and shoulders, for example, simply won't be enough. It is best to try to give a whole body massage where possible. Probably the most sensitive areas will include the abdomen (including the breasts for girls) and the front of the legs. Try beginning with the back — perhaps the least intrusive area, and include the hands and feet before venturing further. Privacy will be important and strict confidentiality essential.

For some of the more serious problems associated with adolescence such as drugs, alcohol and other substance abuse; violence; anorexia; bulimia, and various psycho-sexual disorders, massage can certainly play its part. Obviously though, where a young person may experience disgust with their own body, either through a distorted picture they have of it, or through guilt brought on by sexual abuse of some kind, touch may be the last thing they want or need. In such cases, professional help must be sought and so-called constitutional treatmerrts such as homoeopathy and acupuncture are strongly recommended, as well as the possibility of professional counselling. Professional massage should also be considered since it gives young people the 'space' to express themselves to another in confidence outside the complicated dynamics of the home environment.

Exercise

Adolescence is a period often associated with a great deal of physical exercise. This is a totally normal and quite essential feature of healthy development of mind and body. In fact, it has been noticed that at particular times of stress or anxiety, teenagers may become almost obsessed with physical activity. One reason for this is that it does help regulate and balance some of the excessive sex drive brought on by hyperactive hormones. In any event, as long as exercise doesn't become an obsession in itself, it is clearly a healthy means of dealing with this intense and demanding growth period.

Bach flower remedies

Depression:	Sweet chestnut Gorse
Lack of confidence, feeling inferior:	Larch
Feeling unattractive, ugly:	Crab apple
Anorexia nervosa, bulimia, resentment, feeling isolated and alienated from parents:	Willow
Unsure of which career to pursue/path to follow:	Wild oat
Submissive, failing to speak up for oneself, allowing oneself to be used, perhaps bullied:	Centaury
Lack of enthusiasm, lack of interest:	Gentian
Pre-exam nerves:	White chestnut, Larch, Hornbeam

Crab apple is also beneficial for acne, when applied directly to the skin. Dilute a few drops in a cup of water and bathe the area with it.

Oils

It is most important to allow young people to select the oils whose aroma appeals to them most.

Acne
Bergamot, Lavender, Camomile, Geranium — can be used as a massage oil. Apply morning and evening after washing. Can also be used in a steam inhalation twice a week.

Depression
Bergamot, Rosemary, Basil, Clary sage, Rose,

Jasmine — use in massage; baths; handkerchief inhalation.

Anorexia nervosa
Bergamot, Clary sage, Rose, Neroli, Ylang-ylang — the use of essential oils alone is not enough to treat this condition but when combined with massage, can offset some of the depression and anxiety associated with anorexia nervosa. Use also in baths and in handkerchief inhalation.

Exam nerves
Basil, Rosemary in a bath. Basil and Rosemary have a stimulating effect on the mind and memory so are very useful for long periods of study and during exams. Use also in handkerchief inhalation.

Massage

Back sequence
Have the receiver lying face down and cover them with a towel or blanket. Tuck towel or blanket into underwear. Kneel alongside them facing forward.

1) Make contact (*fig. 167*).

2) Apply the oil to your hands and begin to effleurage from the lower back up onto and across the shoulders. Pull hands back, along the side of torso to the lower back. Repeat at least 15 times.

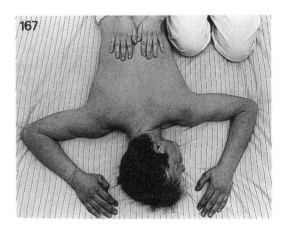

123

3) Come up on knees. Lean hands, fingers facing in opposite directions, alongside spine, heels of hands nearest to spine. Breathe in and as you breathe out lean body weight into hands and push down across the sides of the back. (*fig. 168*) Repeat and continue up entire back.

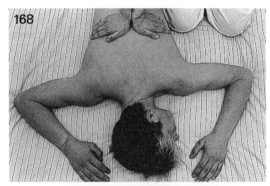

4) Lean thumbs into and along either side of spine; keep whole hands in contact but lean body weight into thumbs (*fig. 169*). Change your position to wide knees alongside the body.

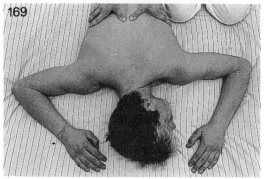

5) Knead, wring, and pull along both sides of the back (*figs. 170, 171 and 172*). To reach the far side of the back, lean up and over your knees.

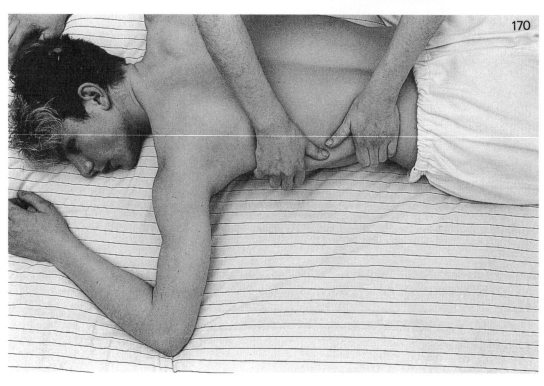

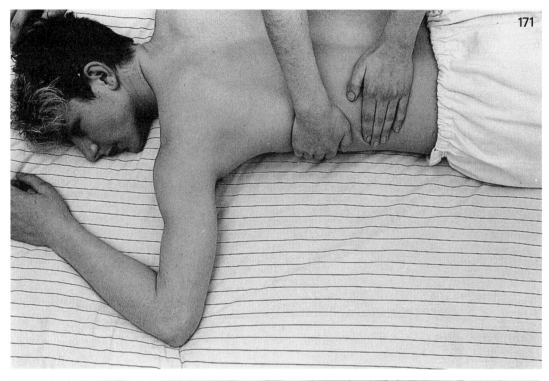

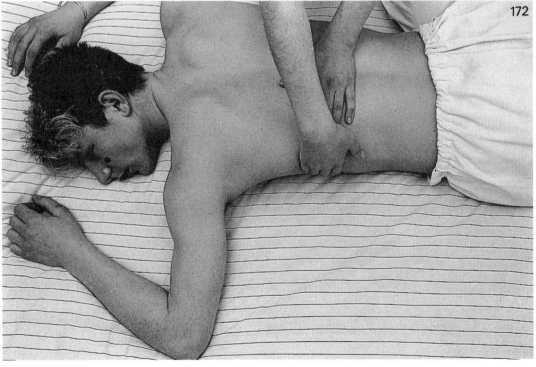

6) Move your body further up, nearer your friend's shoulders. Rest one hand on the upper back and lean the other into and up your friend's neck. Make sure their head is turned away from you (fig 173). Lean your body weight into your hand and squeeze as you come up to the base of the skull (fig. 174).

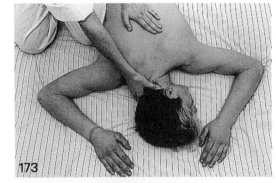

7) Use both hands to squeeze and knead the shoulder muscle (fig. 175). Lean heels and then thumbs into upper back and push up and over the top of the shoulders (figs. 176 and 177). Move to other side and repeat 5 and 6 on other side. Then move astride the head.

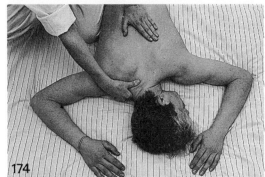

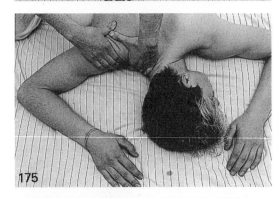

8) Effleurage down the back; bring your body up and over the back as your hands glide down. As your hands come back up to the shoulders, push them alternately into the top of the shoulders (fig. 178).

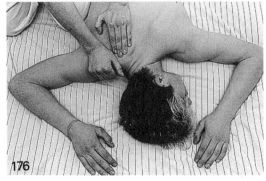

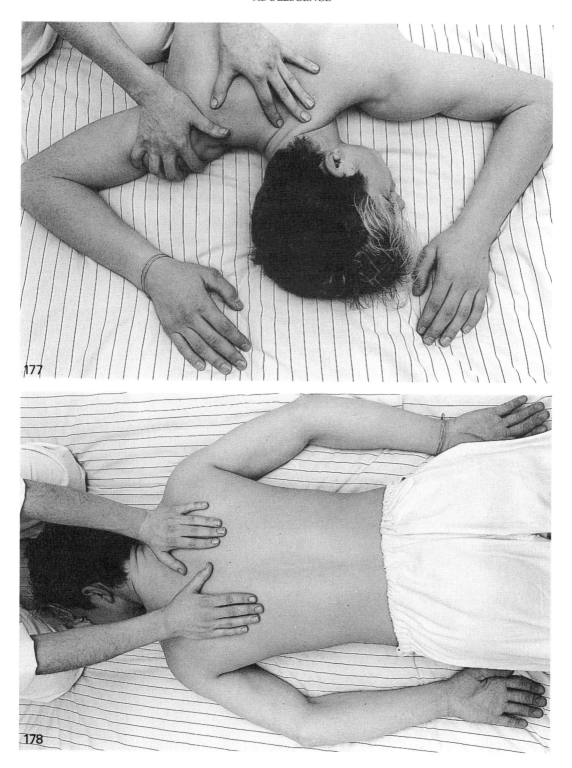

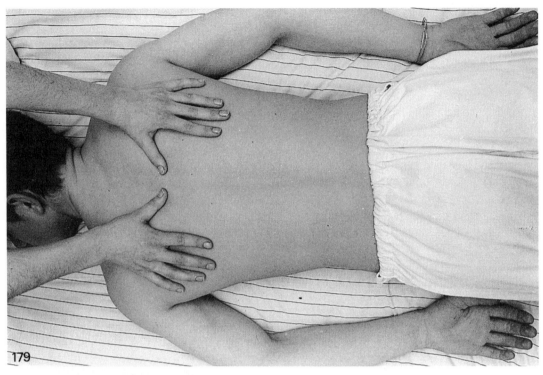

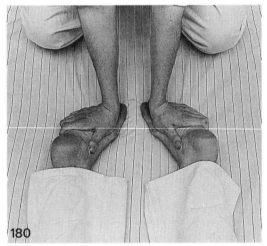

Self-esteem

- I love and accept myself right now. I am good enough at everything I do.
- I am a strong, attractive young woman/ man.
- People love to be with me.
- My presence is a joy to everyone.
- I like and approve of myself in the presence of others.
- I am highly pleasing to myself in the presence of others.
- I am safe and secure.
- I am wonderful as I am.
- I am loving and loveable.

9) Lean thumbs into and along either side of the spine, keeping whole hands in contact (fig. 179).

10) Complete with more effleurage.

11) Stroke the legs and hold the feet (fig. 180).

9

Later life

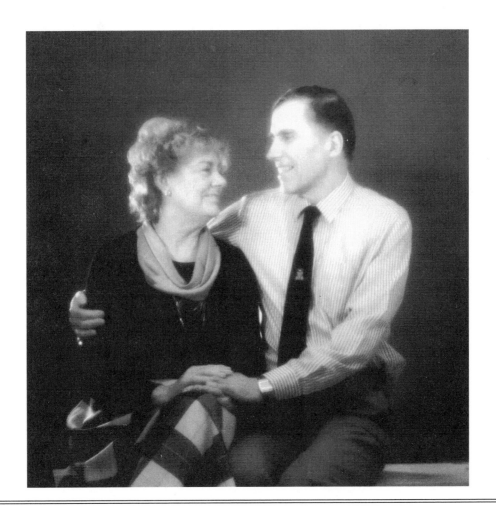

This chapter is entitled Later Life in order to distinguish 'decline of health' from 'old age'. Decline of health is a process that takes place as a result of neglect, lack of exercise, poor diet and abuse of our healthy and mental conditioning. Good health is not a prerogative of youth and nor does it inevitably disappear with increasing years. However, in our Western culture 'old age' has become synonymous with ill-health and withdrawal from active life. Ageing has become the most convenient and widely-accepted excuse for not taking responsiblity for our well-being. Ageing is neither a natural process nor inevitable. Good health is a result of taking care of ourselves, physically, mentally and emotionally and continually investing in it throughout our life, never taking it for granted.

Society has very fixed attitudes about the ageing process. We talk of 'retirement' and decline and the general sense of growing old as one of decreased activity and lessened involvement in life. In modern technological society especially, later life is feared as the break-up of the nuclear family. Fewer pensions have led to an insecurity about material comfort when one ceases to work. There is a fear of being used up, of being left on the shelf, both by one's family and by society as a whole.

The Skin

The skin, which determines much of our ability to adapt to changing circumstances, can show the most visible evidence of poor health: wrinkled, dry and inflexible, it can become the very symbol of what old age means to many of us. Through lack of exercise and neglect, tactile sensitivity is vastly reduced. And yet, because of bereavement and isolation, older people's need to touch and be touched is probably stronger than ever.

It is interesting to note that a huge percentage of individuals die within 18 months of retirement, and within six months after the death of a spouse. It would seem that close companionship and fulfilling a social role through our work are major life supports. Without them our will to live is severely tested. At times of crisis like these in our lives we need to acknowledge the loss and begin to ensure that our emotional and social needs are met in other ways.

Tender, loving human contact can be a powerful substitute for the sexual contact which may gradually diminish in later life. It can help with providing support and comfort to counter the feelings of bitterness and resentment which are too often a feature of growing old and poor health, looking back critically over one's life.

Our particular Western culture has come up with the figure of 70 as the average life span we can expect. This is a totally arbitrary figure and conflicts with cultures whose life expectancy may be quite different. We are all deeply conditioned into associating age with health and energy levels and social activity. We need to guard against holding limiting and destructive thoughts about our bodies, our health and our abilities.

In the past, age has been traditionally associated with wisdom. The so-called sages of China were automatically respected for their experience of life and their advice much sought after. The sayings of Confucius still permeate Chinese society today. Even in modern Japan, company management structure is based on the principle of seniority defined by age, not necessarily by performance or ability. Older people are looked up to, respected and their needs cared for. Naturally, some of this is due to a very sound family unit in societies where grandparents play a vital role and where three generations or more live under the same roof. Nevertheless it is striking to notice to what extent we in the West have developed a singularly unhealthy attitude towards growing old and towards older people in our society.

This is clearly not the case elsewhere in the world and we would do well to re-evaluate this tendency and investigate its origins. Certainly a profound fear of dying seems to afflict many Judaeo-Christian cultures. It is apparently not so rooted in Buddhist, Hindu or Muslim societies. In fact, the mystical image of the Holy Man, whether Yogi, Monk or wandering master is one of a wise ascetic transcending death itself and remaining forever youthful and healthy.

Clearly, our attitude to old age, and the material and pyschological preparations we make for it bind us to a future which holds little hope for us in terms of our quality of life. We have accepted an image of growing old which limits us to a dull, inactive lifestyle which can only compound any physical or emotional disturbances we may feel at this time of great change in our lives. Is it any wonder that, along with these negative thoughts we have about growing old, our body experiences all kinds of painful and debilitating ailments? Research is beginning to link poor self-esteem and negative emotions such as anger, guilt or resentment with diseases like cancer and arthritis. If we equate old age with slowing down and 'retiring' from active life, is it surprising that we should experience bodily aches, pains and stiffness as well as heart problems?

Suddenly stopping work after many years and the possibility of sudden bereavement after a lifetime of companionship may create a vacuum that can cause intense anxiety and depression. One thing is clear. Growing old in society today can be a daunting prospect. Yet it needn't be. With a positive attitude, a healthy diet and plenty of exercise, along with a supportive environment that must include a lot of warmth and touch, we can look forward to future years with anticipation and excitement. Life surely can only get more fulfilling with each new experience and as we get older we may enjoy the added satisfaction of contributing this experience to others, younger than ourselves. We must rediscover the value and privilege of age and

learn to respect it. We take it for granted that age bestows quality and value to things like furniture, wine and even vintage cars! Yet when it comes to human life we somehow forget this. We must focus less on the concept of time itself and more on the character and quality of life as we experience it. We are indeed as 'young as we feel'.

Rigid influences

Too many influences in our lives — families, work, the media, even religion, politics and economics — are geared towards a rigid, fixed interpretation of age and its significance. The person you marry, whether you have children, who your friends are, what you do — even what you believe is easily governed by society's attitude to age.

We are going to examine specific ways in which touch and related therapies may help towards dealing with these issues. But it is worth noting that only when we completely alter the way we look at the process of 'ageing' and free ourselves from some of the absurd preconceptions can we hope to move forward to a brighter, happier and more vital future, both for ourselves and our planet.

We need to acknowledge the possibility that we can all enjoy perfect physical health and youthfulness for the duration of our life. Good health and vitality are clearly not a prerogative of those in their twenties or thirties. It is the product of caring for ourselves, preventative healthcare and a positive mental outlook. Health is clearly a function of participation in life and we all have something to participate in and contribute regardless of our age. Later life is a complex stage of our lives which can be a time of great fulfilment and reward or a time of regret and loneliness. Our experience depends to a large extent on how we evaluate our life to date on the degree of companionship and loving contact we have around us.

Our ideas and beliefs about later life will also shape our experience of it. We live in a culture which sees 'old age' as a time of decay and redundancy, fraught with a succession of any number of ailments which we decide are part of the natural ageing process. Once we decide an ailment is natural and inevitable, we tend not to do anything about it, and abdicate responsibility for its alleviation. Old age and 'ageing' can be the excuse for just about anything from a physical condition to feeling unhappy and despondent about our life.

Senility

At present older people generally receive very little physical contact from the outside world. It is no wonder that many of them shrink and retreat into their own worlds. This is particularly true if their spouse has died and their families are no longer connected to them or live near. Even in older relationships, physical intimacy may no longer be a part of their relationship: so touch *per se* may have been severely reduced. This is also an assumption about ourselves and our libidos that needs challenging. The common complaints that older people take to their doctor are anxiety, depression, lack of energy, arthritis, heart complaints and general aches and pains. Anxiety and depression and lack of energy are largely a result of the extent of aliveness and contentment we experience in our everyday lives. As human beings, we thrive on challenges and goals to aim for. Otherwise our lives may feel humdrum, and lack direction and purpose. If our lifetime employment is no longer available we may need to invent visions and goals. The great sadness is that our culture and many older people forget this. Our society does not value older people as experienced and wise.

In fact we need to change our language completely in order to transform our understanding of this stage in life. 'Experienced' and 'wise' people have an enormous contribution to make to society as a whole while 'old people' suggests a burden and drain (indeed we are often reminded how the increased population of older people is draining health resources in terms of care and medication). It is in contributing to others, and having a purposeful life, that we live life to the fullest. If we deny ourselves new challenges and stimulation we are no longer living fully. There are only two ways of experiencing ourselves: one is to live fully with a commitment to aliveness, and the other is to give up living.

A lot of our disdain and lack of respect for older people comes from the fear we have of stepping into the old age category we have created in our culture. A lot may also come from a deep-seated fear of death. If we see death as something final, an end to life itself, then it appears as a monstrous threat. If we could see it as other world cultures see it, as a renewal, a moving on (with the process of life itself being eternal and immortal) then we might also feel very different about this stage of life. Here again, we need to change language in order to transform our appreciation of this transition.

Instead of the label death, with all its inherent connotations, we could use the word 'renewal', with its connotations of moving on and recharging. We could see ourselves as beings with an essential life-force which can never be extinguished: and has infinite possibilities for re-creation and renewal. The philosphy we hold has the power to open up our life to limitless life and possibilities; or deaden it with fear, worry and limitation.

Massage and Shiatsu

Massage therapies are an ideal way to enhance the quality of life for older people and help avoid, as well as alleviate, many of the common problems they may experience. These will often include stiffness and pain in the joints (arthritis and rheumatism); muscular fatigue and cramps; poor digestion and elimination; general fatigue; depression and anxiety, as well as malfunctions of the internal organs, especially the heart. Hands-on contact is very reassuring as well as calming and relaxing, and may be the only physical communication a single or widowed older person may experience. The physiological benefits of regular massage or shiatsu have been discussed but in particular their ability to improve circulation as well as flexibility of muscles and joints is significant in benefiting older people. Massage, especially with the old, will help keep the skin healthy and full of lustre, whilst shiatsu is particularly good for restoring energy. Both therapies will improve internal secretions. This affects not only digestion but also hormonal balance, which will help stabilize emotional states.

It is possible that older people may not be able to lie on the floor comfortably. It is probably best to concentrate your touch on areas that are easily accessible and which can affect the whole body such as the hands, feet and face. Probably the neck, shoulders and back should also be included.

It will be important to remember certain key factors when working on older people. Make sure the room is warm. (Keep their clothes on.) Sitting in a chair is usually most comfortable and is recommended. All of the massage outlined will assume the person is sitting in a chair. Keep pressure light and gentle. Keep treatment time short. Obviously, certain precautions are also necessary.

○ Don't massage joints locally when inflamed.
○ Don't do any vigorous stretching or manipulation.
○ Get professional advice regarding any serious cardiac disease before massaging.
○ Exercise unaffected joints to improve affected areas.
○ Don't try to exercise affected areas too much.

Massage
Hands Effleurage the hand. Support on cushion. Rotating thumb pressure over back of hand including wrist (*fig. 181*). Heels of palms on back of hand, fingers on palm and smooth over the hand.

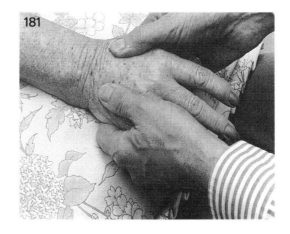
181

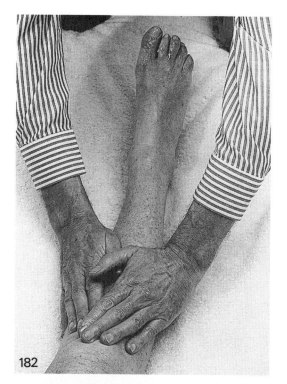

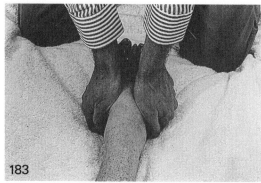

183

182

Feet Make contact. Effleurage up knee (*fig. 182*) over outside foot and leg 20 times. Fingers under sole of foot, heels of palms on top opening the foot out (*fig. 183*). Squeeze across sole of foot. Thumb leaning in and rotating over entire foot (*fig. 184*) including the ankle. In between strokes, stroke over the foot. Rotating thumb on sole of foot and knuckling over top of foot (*fig. 185*) and around ankle. Same on sole (*fig. 186*).

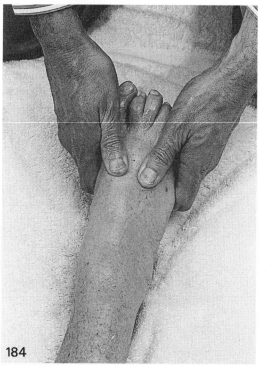

184

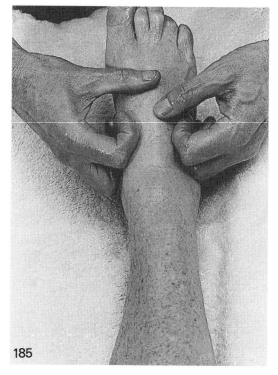

185

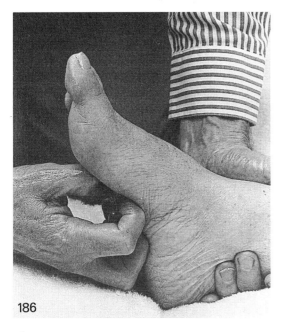

186

Shiatsu

Hands Our hands are our principal tools of work, play and overall activity in life. When we cannot move them freely, we feel inhibited and frustrated. Keeping them flexible and strong is essential to the working of the whole body and to our experience of life. How often we lose heart and spirit when we cannot do things for ourselves with our hands. This may then affect our general health. Massage and shiatsu are excellent for promoting circulation and flexibility in the hands. Certain areas may also stimulate internal organs according to reflexology and Chinese medicine.

Flexibility and warm-up Sit facing your partner to one side and take their hand in yours. Shake hand from wrist to loosen. Begin with a gentle wrist rotation and stretch using one hand as support and one to make the movement. Good support is essential in avoiding any chance of injury. Next, rotate and stretch the thumb and fingers individually using your thumb and forefinger. Then use both hands to stretch open the palm, tucking your little finger behind and onto the back of the hand, your thumbs stretching open the palm. Shake hands from wrist (*fig. 187*). It is extremely beneficial to massage whole area up to the elbow. Effleurage, including the hand.

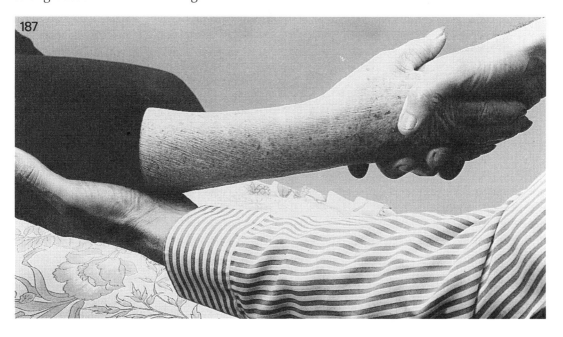

187

Points LI 4 *(fig. 188)* in web of thumb and forefinger — good for general well-being, and locally for arthritis.

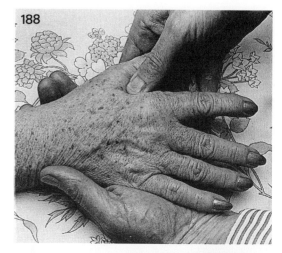

Points in webs of other fingers near knuckles — good for arthritis, stiffness of fingers/poor circulation.

Point in web of 1st and 2nd finger *(fig. 189)* — good for stiff neck.

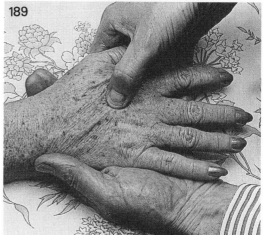

SI 3 *(fig. 190)* on crease formed at side of palm when making a fist — good for stiffness and pain in the back, especially near the spine.

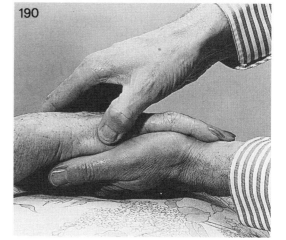

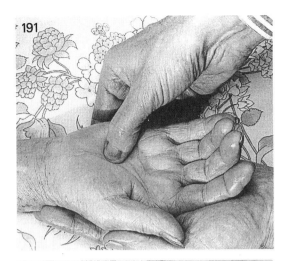

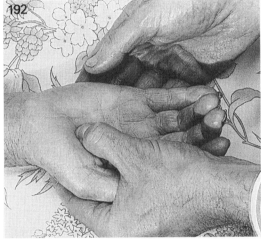

Ht 8/Pe 8 (*fig. 191 and fig. 192*) to stimulate the function of the heart.

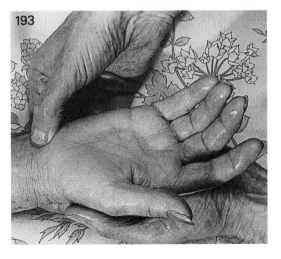

Ht 7 (*fig. 193*) to help alleviate anxiety and depression as well as insomnia which may accompany heart problems.

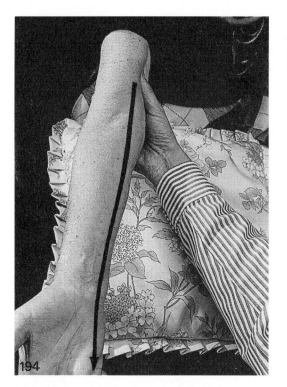

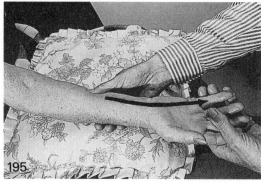

Note: For general heart function, massage along the Ht meridian from under armpits, down inside of arm, little finger side, all the way to the little finger itself (*fig. 194 and 195*). Pull and stretch the finger and pinch the inside corner of the nail (*fig. 196*).

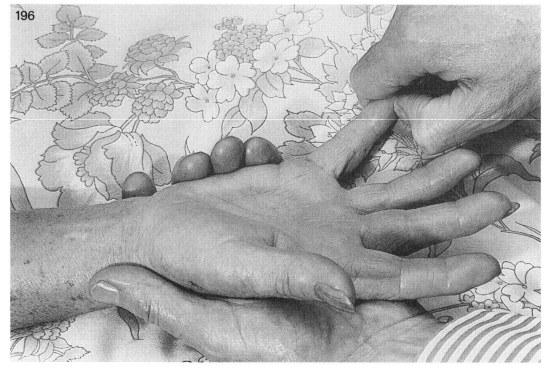

Feet Working on the feet is ideal for older people as it involves the minimum of preparation and movement. Reflexology, or the massage of reflex zones on the foot, has become increasingly popular in recent years, but even without a thorough knowledge of the detailed zones, general massage and shiatsu to the feet can profoundly affect the function of the whole body. Everyone loves to have their feet touched!

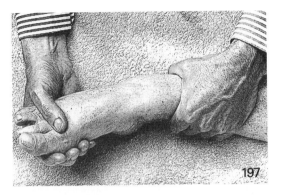

Flexibility and warm-up Sit beside partner's foot, which can be raised onto a stool or your knee. Shake foot from ankle to loosen. As with the hands, rotate and stretch the ankles very slowly both ways using one hand whilst the other supports (*fig. 197*). Rotate and stretch the toes individually using thumb and forefinger (*fig. 198*). Use both hands to stretch the sole of the foot (*fig. 199*). Push thumbs up back of each toe stretching and extending them. Shake foot from ankle to loosen.

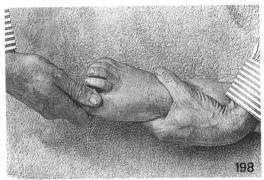

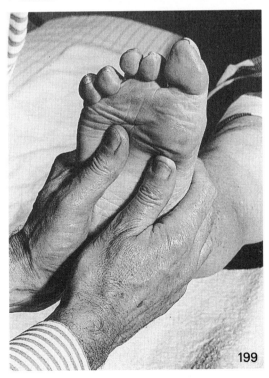

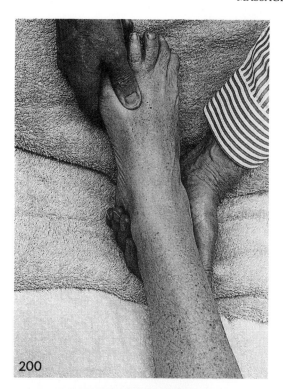

Points Liv 3 *(fig. 200)* — In web between big toe and 2nd toe. Good for regulating liver function.

200

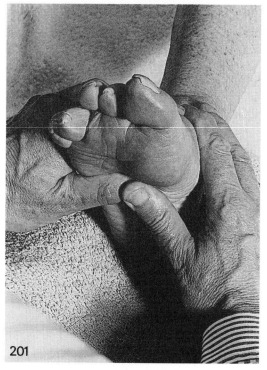

201

Ki 1 *(fig. 201)* — For revitalizing body during recovery from stroke etc.

Ki 3 *(fig. 202)* — For helping fluid metabolism and eliminating water retention.

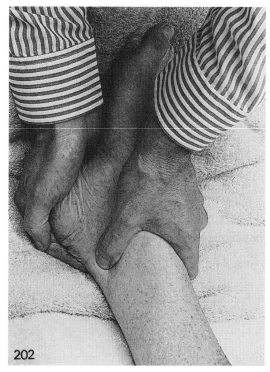

202

UB 60 (*fig. 203*) — For backaches and bladder function.

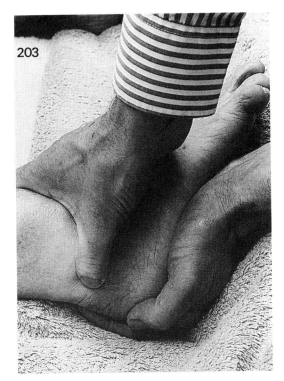

Note: To do specific treatment on the knee, move up alongside knee, stroking whole hand up and over knee joints. Circling thumb movements around kneecap. Then individual thumb movements around kneecap. Shiatsu points as illustrated. St 36 (*fig. 204*) for knee problems and general well-being.

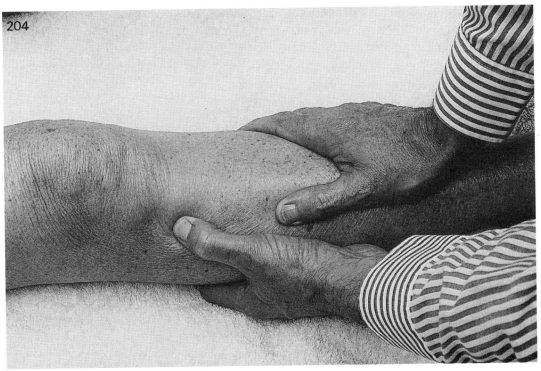

Head, neck, face and shoulders A great deal of premature ageing is often due to tension in the face. Our face reflects the way we think, feel and act, and inevitably, our conclusions about life. Our true thoughts and feelings are indeed 'written all over our face'. The face itself has more muscles than the rest of the body put together and easing tension out of it with soothing massage and shiatsu will relax and revitalize the whole body and ultimately make a difference to the way we see ourselves. A good facial massage will often make a person look five or ten years younger. It's a bit like an unmasking process to reveal your true self and allow it to be expressed.

The face treatment is complete in itself but it is extremely effective when combined with the neck and shoulders. They are the storehouse of stress and tension, and working here is extremely beneficial for the whole body.

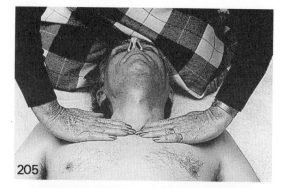

205

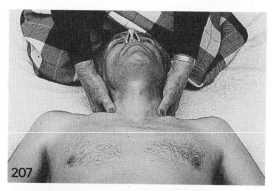

206

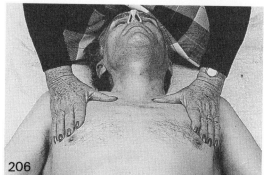

207

Sequence Partner lying on back. Giver kneeling at head. Make contact.

1) Place thumbs, fingers touching, below collar bone on upper chest (fig. 205). Slowly slide hands across chest in opposite directions, under shoulders and up back of neck. Repeat at least five times.

2) Leaving thumbs in between ribs gently moving from centre of chest outwards, as far as nipples (take care when treating women). (fig. 206) One hand holding side of head, other hand leaning in and gently squeezing side and back of neck (fig. 207). Change hands and repeat. Move hand round to front of neck, gentle thumb squeezing to front of neck.

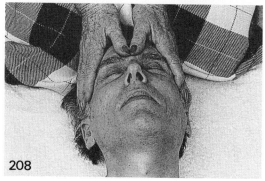

208

Note: Light pressure only! Next one hand supporting shoulder, other hand gently squeezing shoulder muscle between thumb and fingers. Move to face. Make contact on face, thumbs facing nose, fingers resting on sides of head (*fig. 208*). Gentle leaning pressure onto thumbs, sliding them in the following sequence across the face. Keep hands relaxed and in constant contact with skin surface.

Do all lines twice. Forehead — 3 lines across (*figs. 209, 210 and 211*). Eyebrows — from inside to outside and beyond temples (*figs. 212 and 213*). Under eyes — from inside to outside and beyond temples (*fig. 214*). Corner of nose — round cheekbone in front of ears (*figs. 215, 216 and 217*). Upper lip — from sides of nose past corners of mouth down to chin (*fig. 218*). Lower lip — across jaw bone up to ear (*figs. 219 and 220*). Under jaw — finger pressure massage. Ears — squeeze gently and stretch (*fig. 221*).

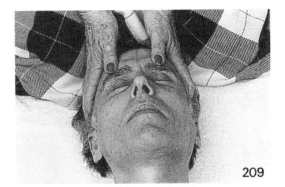

209

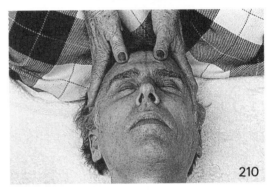

210

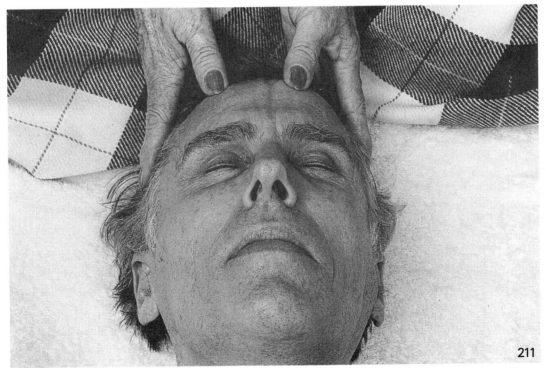

211

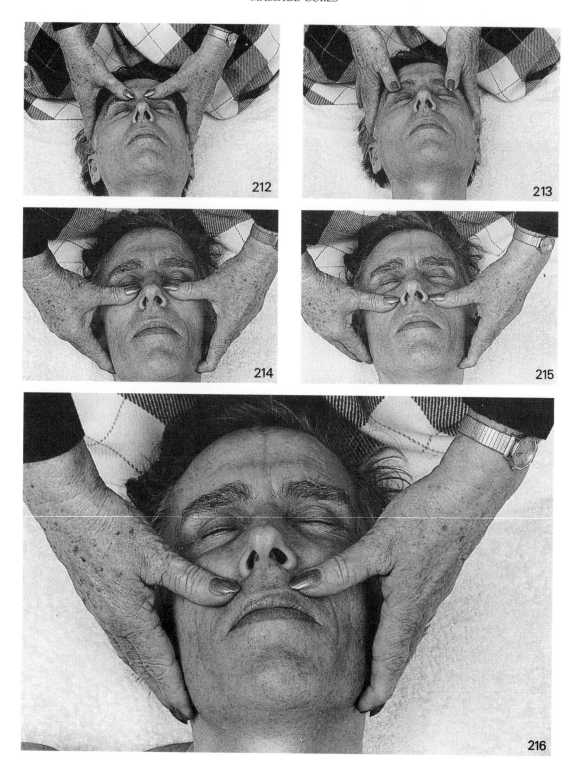

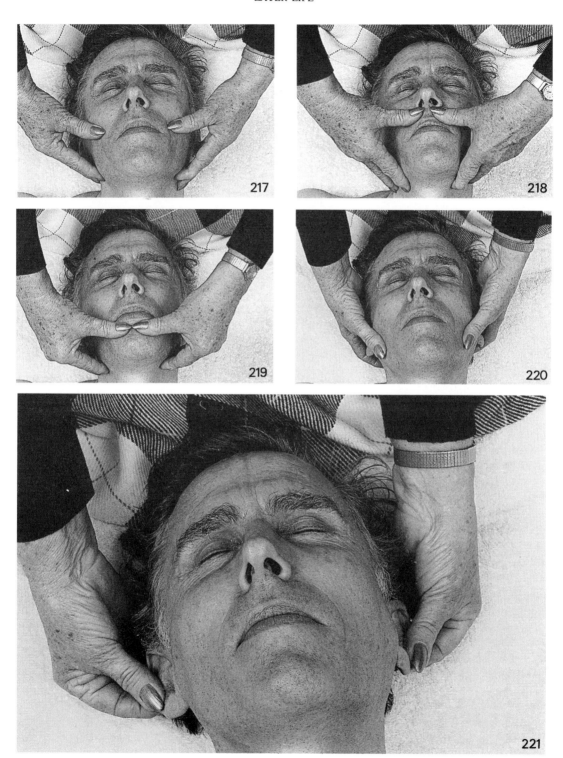

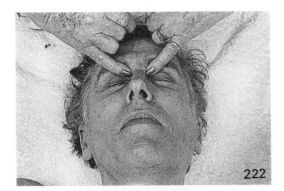

222

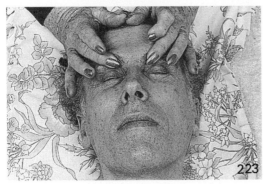

223

Points During massage you may concentrate on the following points: UB 1 (*fig. 222*), UB 2 (*fig. 223*) — Improves eyesight. TH 21 (*fig. 224*) SI 19 (*fig. 225*) — Improves hearing. GV 20 (*fig. 226*) — Clears mind, uplifts and strengthens internal energy.

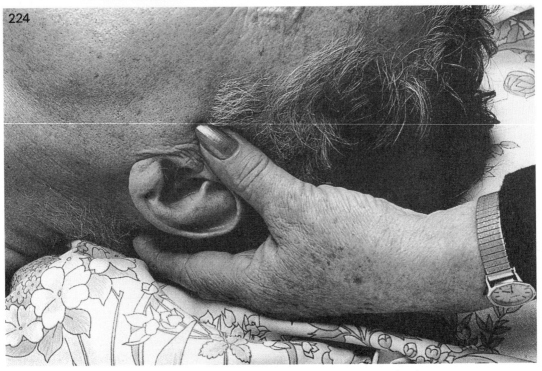

224

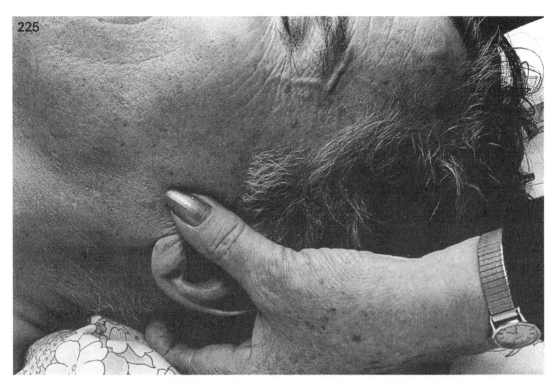

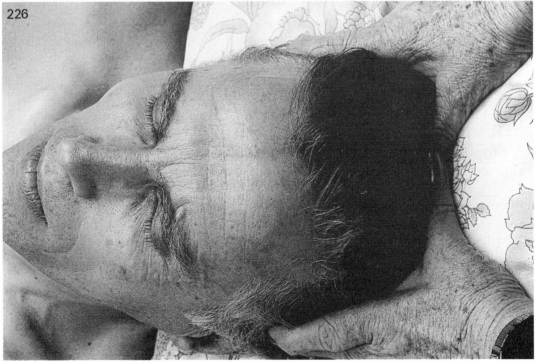

Back The back is often a source of stress and tension in later life. It houses the spinal column which affects the whole body and is part of the central nervous system. It is supported by large muscle groups which, when tense, can easily distort the whole body and create spinal problems. Chronic tension in the back can often cause poor posture, which compounds the problems of pain and inflexibility in the area. Sometimes, in later life, spinal fluids may dry up, causing added stiffness and inflexibility. The back is the single largest area of the body. It holds us up, and its strength and flexibility often reflect the degree to which we feel supported in ourselves and in our lives. Experiencing life as a burden can often be reflected in rounded, drooping shoulders and a stoop as though the person were literally weighed down by a heavy weight.

A good way for an elderly person to receive a back massage is for them to straddle a chair,

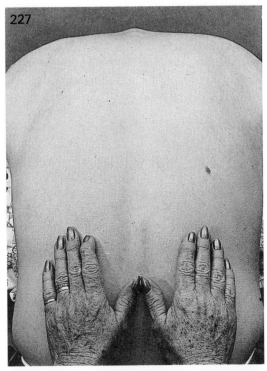

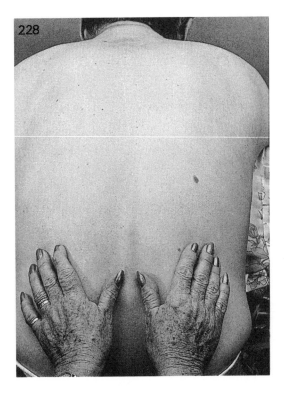

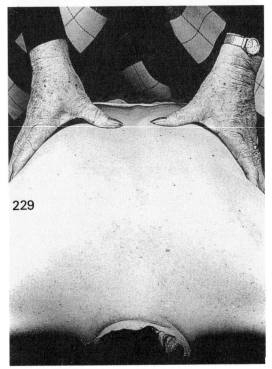

facing the back, using a cushion to keep the front of the body comfortable.

1) Make contact (*fig. 227*).

2) Effleurage entire back from lower to upper (*fig. 228*).

3) Thumbs leaning in and circling alongside spine (*fig. 229*) from lower to upper and up to neck.

Note: Alongside the spine, the acupuncture points have special significance in affecting the internal organs. Points to be used are: UB 15, UB 18, UB 23. See Chapter 6 on pregnancy for back squeeze.

Bach flower remedies

Tiredness/exhaustion:	Olive
Looking to the past, bereavement:	Honeysuckle
Resignation, apathy:	Wild rose
Despondency, lack of interest:	Gentian
Bitterness, resentful:	Willow
Deep depression, anguish, 'what's the use':	Gorse
Inflexible, not willing to see others' point of view:	Vine
Terror, fear, agoraphobic:	Rock rose
Guilt or blaming oneself for the mistakes of others or oneself:	Pine
Forgetfulness, absentmindedness:	Clematis
Anxiety, and fearing the future:	Aspen
Lack of confidence, unable/unwilling to try new things:	Larch

Essential oils

Arthritis is an illness that involves a complex association of factors. It should be treated by a naturopath in order to make dietary changes that will cleanse and strengthen the body. In cases of inflammation, acupuncture may be valuable. However, oils can be useful in stimulating the body's own resources to eliminate toxic buildup in the joints and prevent further buildup.

Massage with oils is most effective. Use Benzoin, Camomile, Cypress, Fennel, Juniper, Lavender, Lemon and Rosemary, Black pepper, Ginger and Marjoram. Combine three of the above in vegetable oil, massage on the affected area and wrap in a warm cover. *Baths* — any of the above oils can be also used in a bath. *Compresses* — the most suitable oils to use in a hot compress are the pain-killing ones such as Lavender, Camomile, Rosemary and Benzoin.

Depression/anxiety — Lavender, Neroli, Bergamot, Geranium, Basil, Rosemary, Rose. Used to have an uplifting effect. *Baths* — use 6-10 drops in any combination of three of the above. *Massage* — the reassuring touch of a caring therapist will enhance the effectiveness of the oils. *Handkerchief inhalation* — apply 2-3 drops of any of the above oils and inhale during the day.

Forgetfulness/poor memory — Basil/Rosemary. *Handkerchief inhalation* — use as above. *Baths* — ideally used in morning time baths or before going out in the evening.

Resignation/apathy — Bergamot, Marjoram, Rosemary, Lavender. *Baths* — these oils are stimulating so are best used in the morning and not at night. *Handkerchief inhalation* — use any of the oils to inhale during the day.

Poor circulation/strengthening the heart — Garlic, Lavender, Marjoram, Peppermint, Rose and Rosemary all have a strengthening effect on the heart muscle. Lavender, Melissa, Neroli and Ylang-ylang are useful for disorders such as palpitations. The use of these oils, especially with massage, can be of great benefit, especially in improving the overall circulation throughout the body. However, a serious heart complaint must always be treated by a qualified practitioner. *Massage* — use any three of the above oils in a vegetable oil. *Baths* — use 6-10 drops in morning or evening bath. Peppermint and Rosemary are best used in a morning bath because they are so stimulating. Use only one drop of Peppermint.

Self-esteem

As mentioned earlier, a healthy mental outlook is essential to our physical well-being and to the life we create for ourselves. With regard to specific physical ailments and their mental counterparts, Louise Hay, in her book *You Can Heal Your Life*, offers specific mental causes and affirmations.

Arthritis: Feeling unloved, criticism, resentful.

○ I am love, I now choose to love and approve of myself.
○ I see others with love.

Heart: Long-standing emotional problems, lack of love. Hardening of the heart. Belief in strain and stress.

○ I lovingly allow joy to flow through my mind and body and experience.

Heart attacks: Squeezing all the joy out of the heart in favour of money and position.

○ I bring joy back to the centre of my heart.
○ I express love to all.

General supportive thoughts that may also help are:

○ My body is getting stronger and fitter every day.
○ My presence is a joy to everyone.
○ I now have enough energy to do everything I want to do.
○ I love and approve of myself completely.
○ I am trusting God/the universe to support me completely.
○ I always have enough money to do everything I want to do.
○ I am a loving, lovable, worthwhile person and I deserve to be loved.

10

Exercise and sport

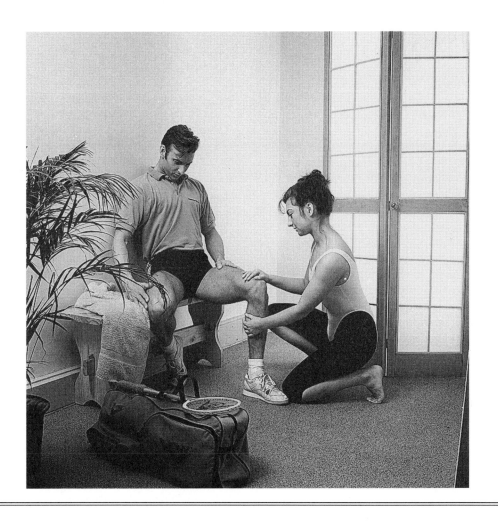

One of the main features of the modern working environment is the gradual move that has taken place from outside to indoors, and from the countryside to the city. With it has come an increasingly sedentary lifestyle where one may retain the same, often cramped and unnatural posture all day with little or no opportunity to exercise. Office or factory work, housekeeping, or school study all expose the body to artificial light and temperature as well as depriving it of movement. We can quickly become unfit, sluggish and easily tired. A vicious circle can easily develop. Under these conditions stress has more chance of producing an adverse effect on the body, which is less able to cope as a result. We may often know we should exercise but just don't feel like it. In fact, the slightest amount of exercise may quickly tire and discourage us.

A sensible routine

It is important to build up an exercise routine slowly. It is always best to be realistic about your level or self-discipline. Choose a work partner or friend to exercise with. You can then support each another: pushing where necessary and congratulating where there is progress. It may be useful to make short- and long-term goals. This gives you a way to measure your achievements.

Prepare a programme for yourself. The initial novelty will inevitably wear off so you will need an incentive to keep going. Monitoring your improvement will boost you when your commitment flags. Measure your achievements (statistics) and use friends as coaches or advisors for those times when your mind starts sending those familiar discouraging thoughts like: 'Is this doing me any good?' 'What's the point?' 'I feel tired', etc. Or create empowering thoughts such as: 'I'll feel 20 years younger after this' or 'When I'm fit, I'm happy and fulfilled'.

Any fit person will tell you of the multiple benefits of regular exercise. One eats, sleeps and generally performs better and with less effort. Physical fitness makes you feel mentally sharper, physically more comfortable, more in tune with your body and better able to cope with the demands of everyday life. You feel alert and full of energy, and at the same time relaxed and contented. Some people even claim to be addicted to exercise which releases endorphins, the natural body 'happy hormones'.

The kind and amount of exercise you do is crucial and may depend on your age, general health and needs. It is advisable to seek professional advice as to the exact requirements of your body given your job, age, diet, sleep pattern and general level of fitness. In the final analysis, however, you are the best judge of what your body needs to keep fit.

It is important to recognize that a clear distinction exists between what we can call internal and external exercise. Your body needs both. In the martial arts practices of the Far East, this distinction has been recognized for thousands of years. Kung Fu, Judo, Karate are all classed as 'external' whilst Tai Chi, Chi-kung, yoga, Ba hua and Shing Yi are all 'internal' martial arts. Meditation is clearly a form of internal exercise and the martial arts are forms of meditation in themselves. Tai Chi is often described as movement meditation.

External exercise is usually dynamic in form, involving intense physical exertion with increased breathing and heart rates and vigorous body movement. It develops the voluntary muscle groups, improving strength and tonus and increases cardio-respiratory fitness. Suppleness and flexibility of the joints is enhanced, the digestive and excretory systems stimulated and one's circulation and general fitness improved. External exercise also improves the production of internal secretions, a major factor in weight loss and pain relief. Internal exercise is apparently more passive when viewed from the outside and relies less on physical movement and exertion. It develops the involuntary muscle groups and improves homoeostatis in the body. Emphasis is placed on learning to feel and move the more subtle energies in the body in order to balance them. This is done through subtle but disciplined movement and focuses especially on the breathing.

Internal exercise will not only improve energy flow but also increase the amount of energy available within the body. Its long-term effects are to enhance one's powers of concentration, producing clear, disciplined thinking as well as a feeling of calm and contentedness. Internal exercise provides the necessary base upon which to build external strength and fitness. It is important for the body to be strong and robust in order to resist disease and to be supple and flexible to adapt to life's ever-changing rhythms. The true aim of all the martial arts was originally this subtle combination of outer strength and inner softness both of which provide the key to health, happiness and longevity.

Growth of the health club

Exercise and fitness are now popular pursuits where once they were the domain of professional sports people and athletes. In the last 20-30 years we have seen a phenomenal boom in the health and fitness industry. Fitness is now a major growth industry and health clubs are unrecognizable from the traditional athletes' gym. They are now luxurious social centres where we can include exercise as an enjoyable way of spending our social and leisure time. Health clubs may well be fast becoming the singles bars of the nineties where we can be sure to meet like-minded, exercise-minded people. The fitness craze may change and fluctuate in particular trends, but there is no doubt that it is here to stay.

This tremendous upsurge in exercise participation has brought with it specific demands and problems. The high-impact aerobics craze in the USA and throughout the world led to a universal catalogue of aerobics injuries and strains. Through trial and error we have learned the pitfalls of some of the newer forms of exercise and modified them accordingly. High-impact aerobics has become low-impact aerobics and the popularity of jogging suffered a severe setback with the death of its great advocate, Jimmy Fixx.

Jimmy Fixx took up jogging when he was in his fifties and became famous for popularizing jogging as the answer to modern health problems especially heart disease. His untimely death at the age of 54 surprised the exercise world and forced the realization that vigorous exercise was not necessarily the modern panacea it had been thought to be.

Exercise is essential to a healthy body and mind: however there are other equally essential ingredients. A well-balanced diet will support your body, especially when you have increased demands on it in an exercise programme.

Perhaps most important is providing deep rest and recuperation for your body. When we take vigorous exercise we stimulate the sympathetic nervous system which activates the responses and energy necessary to carry out this exercise. To balance this stimulation we need to involve the parasympathetic nervous system. This system provides for balance and relaxation and regeneration within the body. These two opposite, yet complementary, modes of energy can be compared to the left and right functions of the brain: the right more passive and meditative, the left more active and energetic. For both the mind and the body, to achieve optimum health we need to strike a balance. In terms of exercise, we need to balance aerobic exercise with slow stretching and strength work.

Indeed, we actually need to create an individual balance for ourselves regardless of current trends. It helps if it is relevant to our personality and lifestyle. The stressed executive who works in a highly competitive environment may be drawn to competitive sports like squash: but to achieve balance in his life and profound benefit from his exercise, he would be much better to prioritize a more relaxing activity such as yoga or Tai Chi. His sympathetic nervous system is already overstressed and his parasympathetic is probably not being mobilized to allow relaxation and recuperation. Balance in our lives and our exercise must be the criteria when choosing an exercise programme.

The correct motivation in performing exercise is extremely important. Many of us resort to exercise in an attempt simply to lose weight, and the exercise becomes only about losing weight. Exercise *is* important for losing weight and gaining health; however, there is the danger that we may grow to dislike and dread our chosen exercise if it only ever reminds us that we still need to lose weight and improve our body. We need to see exercise as a permanent feature in our lives and not as a temporary weight reduction technique. The human body is an extraordinary, irreplaceable machine that needs to be regularly and consistently exercised to function at its best. It is the only machine that actually improves with use and decays through lack of use. Our bodies are meant to carry us through life in an active way. Therefore we need to choose exercise that we actually enjoy

doing and regard as an essential part of looking after ourselves. We also need to develop greater acceptance of our bodies as they are now: rather than despising them until they're different.

There is a great tendency with exercise goals and aims to put off feeling good about our bodies until they've achieved certain measurements. It is interesting to notice if we blame our bodies for not having achieved what we think we should have in other areas of our life. If we are feeling not good enough about ourselves we may project this onto our bodies and blame them! This creates a vicious circle where we get stuck in only ever seeing our bodies in a negative light.

The way we see our bodies affects our physical shape. If we only ever see ourselves as overweight and ungainly then we are creating an overweight and ungainly future for ourselves! This is creative visualization at its most basic level. We need to see our bodies as gaining health and vitality every day, whilst at the same time not denying them as they are now. Also, it can happen that our bodies have made progress and developed but we fail to notice! Anorexia sufferers see themselves as huge and amorphous even though they may be near starvation and weigh only 70-75 pounds.

Routines

Daily exercise of one hour or more is recommended to include both internal and external exercises. Warming up for either type of exercise is essential.

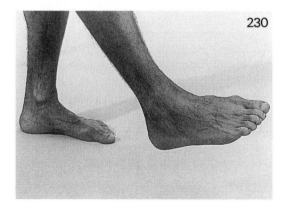

230

Warm-up: done from foot to head
1) Shake foot at ankle — rotate (*fig. 230*).

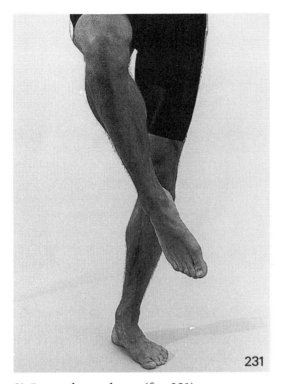

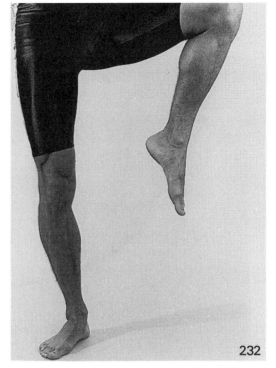

231

232

2) Rotate leg at knee (*fig. 231*).

3) Circle hip (*fig. 232*).

4) Stretch calves/hamstrings/rectus femoris (muscle at the front of the thigh) (*fig. 233, 234 and 235 respectively*).

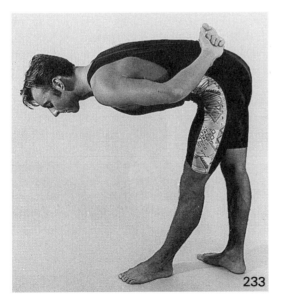

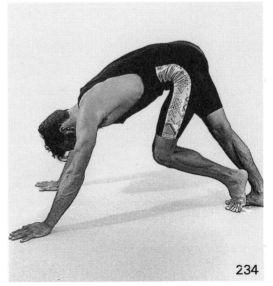

233

234

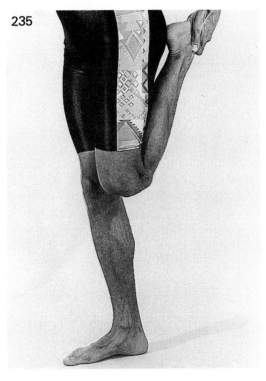

235

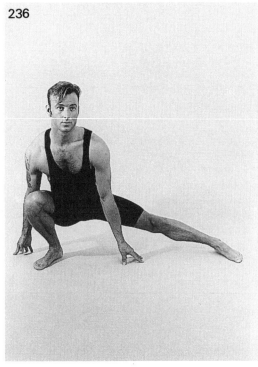

236

5) Lunge to side, one leg bent, one straight, stretching inside of legs and opening groin area (*fig. 236*).

6) Squatting and stomach stretch (*figs. 237, 238 and 239*).

7) Hands interlinked — circle trunk left to right (*figs. 240 and 241*).

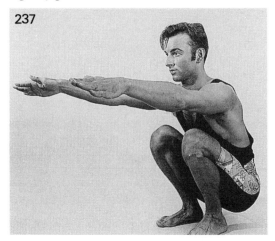

237

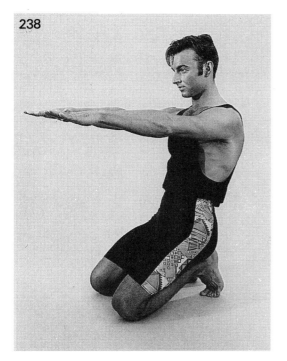

238

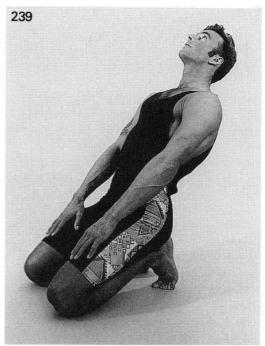

239

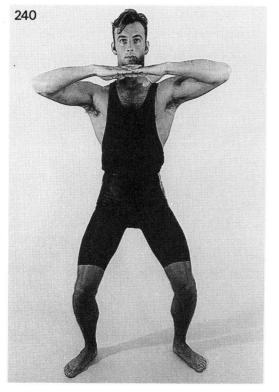

240

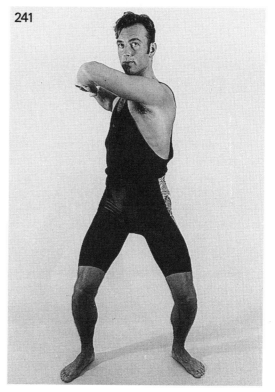

241

157

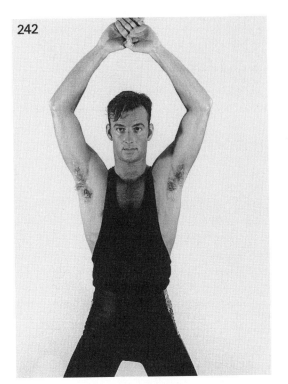

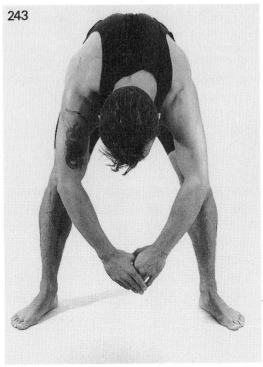

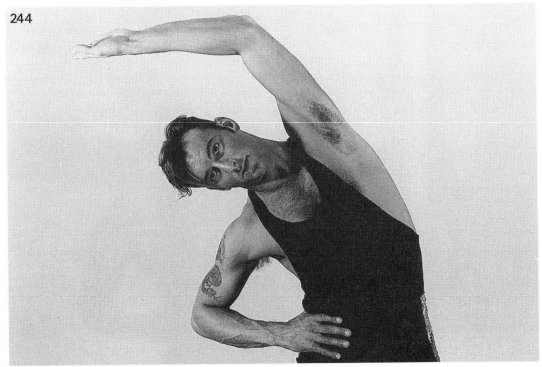

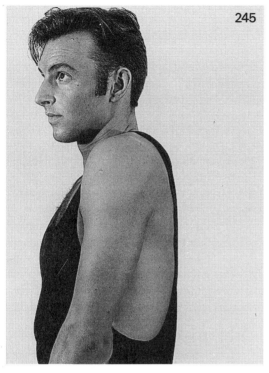

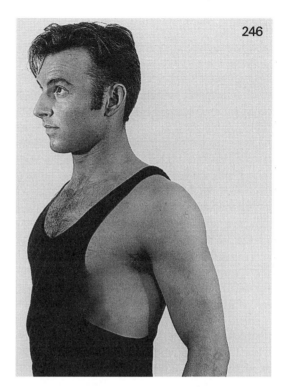

8) Hands interlinked — swing hands down etc (*figs. 242 and 243*).

9) Rest one hand on waist. Lean to side, taking arm over head. Stretch with legs bent (*fig. 244*).

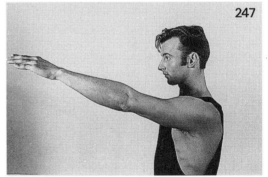

10) Circle point of shoulders each side. Both ways/together (*figs. 245 and 246*).

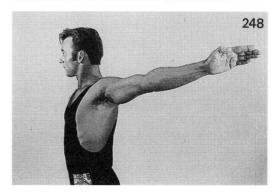

11) Circle arm at shoulder each side. Both ways/together (*figs. 247 and 248*).

249

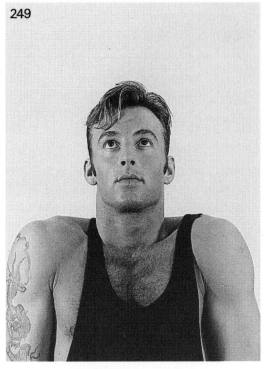

250

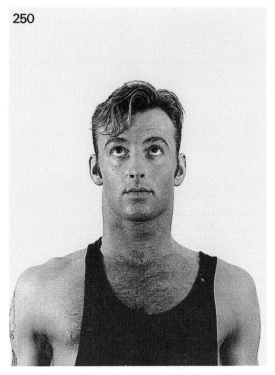

251

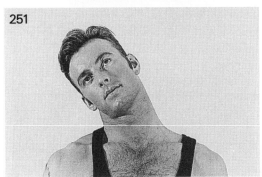

12) Raise shoulders to ears, and drop (*figs. 249 and 250*).

13) Neck movements: Side to side; front to back; ear to shoulders (*figs. 251, 252, 253 and 254*).

252

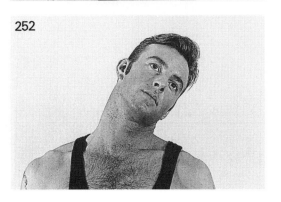

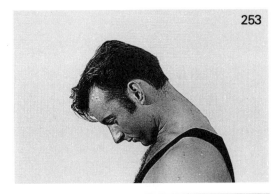

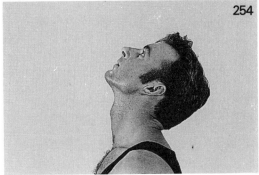

14) Eye movements: up/down; left/right; clockwise; anticlockwise (*figs. 255, 256, 257 and 258*).

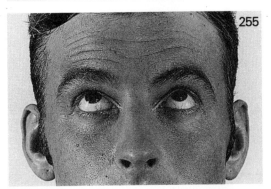

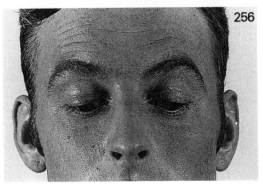

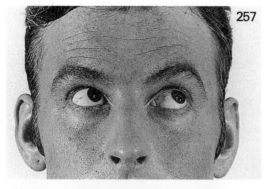

257

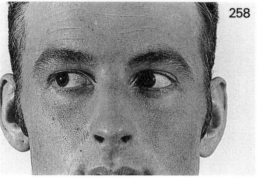

258

The above sequence can be used as a form of exercise in its own right and is an ideal five-minute whole body tone-up, at work or when time and space is limited.

External exercise

It is important to go to a gym and receive proper qualified instruction which gives incentive and healthy criticism to your progress. Exercises as suggested by a fitness consultant should include: aerobics, including cycling/rowing/jogging/swimming; press ups/sits ups (ten times each); weight training (light weights and high repetition); rebounding; skipping; stretch exercises.

Internal exercises

Often these are best done after a full day at work and can allow you to let off steam or unwind after the pressures of the day. Ideally, you should attend classes on a regular basis. You may choose yoga, of which there are various forms or styles, some more dynamic than others, or Tai Chi, a Chinese movement system originally a martial art but often practised simply for health. Thousands of people practise it each morning in parks through-out China. Chi Kung, from which Tai Chi probably originally evolved, is a more static but extremely powerful method of internal energy development, concentrating on posture and breathing. Do-in Ankyo is a Japanese exercise, meditation and self-treatment system, less well-known in this country but incorporating elements of Oriental medical theory designed to balance and regulate the energies of the body to give good health. It involves a comprehensive system of spiritual and physical exercise, meditation and self-massage. Forms of meditation which are ideal internal exercises include a variety of Oriental systems like TM; Taoist and Tibetan meditation and esoteric yoga.

One or more of these 'soft' martial arts is an ideal way to focus on your breathing and to learn to centre yourself (fig. 259). Finding a good teacher who inspires you is important. Patience and commitment are essential ingredients to gaining the benefits of prac-

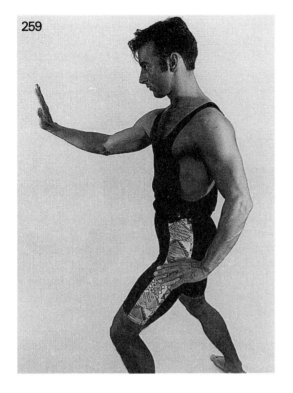

259

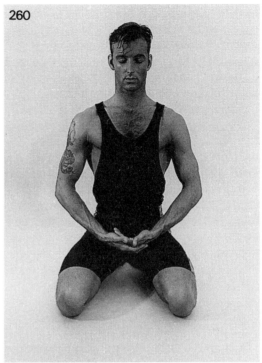

260

tice. It usually takes a good deal longer to notice the subtle changes within the mind and body produced by internal exercise as opposed to the more obvious immediate benefits of external exercise. Generally, the more dynamic internal exercises like yoga or Tai Chi are best done in the early morning before work.

Meditation is often done first thing and last thing in the day, to begin and complete your waking hours (fig. 260). It is interesting to notice that the systems of exercise of the East and West have evolved very differently and have distinct characters. Oriental exercise systems certainly pre-date treatment systems such as acupuncture, moxibustion, and herbal medicine and were probably the first forms of preventative medicine. They work on the body's energy system, both externally and internally, balancing the whole person. This translates into flexibility and strength of the muscles, tendons and joints; improved

respiration and circulation; increased internal secretions improving digestion and hormonal balance; enhancing the general well-being of the person making them feel relaxed and revitalized.

In other words, the design of the Oriental exercise systems is to go far beyond the concept of mere 'fitness', towards achieving total health for the whole person, mind and body. In the West we have tended to lay particular emphasis on developing cardio-respiratory fitness, strengthening and toning the muscles or the 'external' body. We have overlooked the importance of 'internal' exercise based on balancing the subtle energies of the body through the more focused meditative and generally softer systems common to the Orient. In short, we have failed to fully exercise the whole person. In Britain, traditional home of team sports, exercise has often been a convenient side-effect of the spirit of competition. Not until Roger Bannister broke the four-minute mile did the concept of exercising by and for oneself really reach the common consciousness. From the post-war period until today, the fitness boom is well known as having produced such practices as keep-fit; aerobics; weight training and jogging.

But it was only really in the last 20 years or so that, as people notice the benefits of exercise in their daily lives, the concept of 'fitness' has expanded to include 'whole health'. With it has come an increased awareness and concern for our body and the environmental factors which affect it. We are more careful now about the food we eat, the water we drink, the air we breathe and the amount of exercise and the medication we take. Organic fruit and veg, natural husbandry of animals, purified water. ionizers, smoke-free zones and exhaust emission reducers, natural medicines: in short the whole 'green' movement is gathering momentum.

Perhaps the most important and endearing feature of all this is that we no longer see ourselves as separate from our bodies or our bodies from our environment. Exercise and developing and keeping in touch with this awareness of our bodies has made this possible.

Massage and Shiatsu

The relationship between sport and massage has a long history. The gladiators of ancient Rome were massaged with oils before combat and today, most professional sports people regularly use massage as an integral part of their training. It's used both for prevention and treatment of injury. Used before physical activity it can improve the flexibility of muscles, preventing adhesions and reducing the risk of strain or sprain. It increases circulation and lymphatic flow which helps in oxygen exchange, respiratory performance as well as in clearing lactic acid buildup in the muscles which can cause cramps and stiffness. It can also drastically reduce recovery

times as well as help prevent stiffness and soreness following exercise.

Muscles often contract and shorten after exercise, especially running, and this can reduce flexibility and elasticity. Regular massage is the best way to treat this situation. Many forms of massage are used specifically to treat tissue injury, though it is advisable to seek professional help in such cases. Physiotherapy has traditionally been seen as the sports injury treatment of preference, though acupuncture and moxibustion, acupressure and shiatsu as well as massage (by professionally qualified practitioners) are all thoroughly recommended. For minor injuries including sprains and strains, providing you have checked for any complications like hairline fractures etc. first with a professional, you can safely try some of the techniques below. **Note:** Massage can help us accept our bodies as they are now, as opposed to feeling cut off from them until we have made certain physical 'improvements'.

The fitness boom may have peaked and some of the evidence of over-exercise may be all too apparent. But activities like jogging, weight training and aerobics are as popular as ever and the importance of simple, easily-performed massage strokes pre- and post-exercise are an essential part of keeping fit and healthy. Regular massage teaches us to balance exercise with relaxation. Balance is really the key to understanding and developing our minds and bodies.

In weight training, if we do not develop muscles evenly, imbalance will occur, creating postural imbalance and increasing the risk of injury. The same applies in our whole approach to exercise. If we do not balance periods of intense exercise and activity with moments of peace and relaxation such as during massage, we may find such efforts ultimately counterproductive. Too much exercise with nothing to balance it may simply end up compounding the very stresses and tensions which we are trying to remove. They may become locked into the body. Massage is an ideal way of releasing such tension before it accumulates and creates postural imbalances.

In giving massage it is important to include deep stroking (see Chapter 2) to cover the whole muscle. This spreads the invididual fibres and increases circulation as well as eliminating metabolic by-products. Also, cross-fibre strokes (kneading across the muscle) will help break adhesions which can easily lead to cramp and injury. It is important to concentrate too on ligaments and connective tissue around joints. Included below are mainly leg sequences as these apply to almost all types of exercise. Refer to Chapter 6 for back massage. We do not include suggestions on compresses for injury here because there are several schools of thought on this subject. Most textbooks suggest cold compresses for sprains etc. in order to reduce swelling. But cold will often stagnate blood in the area locally and slow up the healing process. Other books recommend compresses alternating hot and cold. Sometimes a herb with healing properties like ginger is used in compress form to increase local circulation. You will have to reach your own decision on the effectivenss of each of these methods.

One general rule that does apply is to mas-sage an equivalent area to the size of the injury on the other, unaffected side of the body. In shiatsu, this is done because there is an obvious link between, for example, the left and right knees, through the meridian system. Treating the one will affect the other and it is naturally easier and less painful to treat the good side first. Strong or insensitive pressure or over-exercise at the site of an injury will cause the whole body simply to tense up and retard the healing process. Equally, where possible, gentle movement of the injured joint is recommended since long-term strapping or immobilizing will impair natural healing. Treatment of injury is the subtle art of generating movement of the joint or muscle as much as possible whilst being careful not to overdo it.

Ankles
The flexibility of the ankles often has a great bearing on the flexibility of the whole body. Because in the West we sit on chairs and not our feet, people's ankles tend to be quite stiff. Ankle sprains or strains can occur just as easily when a person is tired or momentarily loses their concentration as when they are doing strenuous exercise. See Chapter 9 for foot and ankle massage. An alternative sequence would include:

See shiatsu sequence on page 139. Use same points as before but include GB 40 (*fig. 261*), Sp 5 (*fig. 262*), UB 62 (*fig. 263*), Ki 6 (*fig. 264*), St 41 (*fig. 265*) as well as any tender areas around joint and on sole and top of foot.

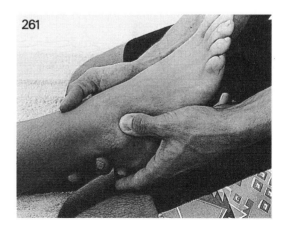

261

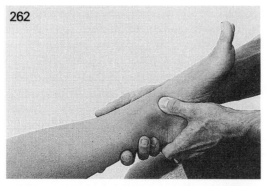

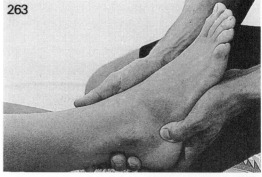

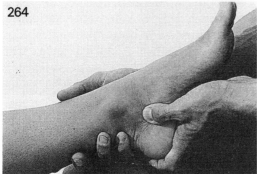

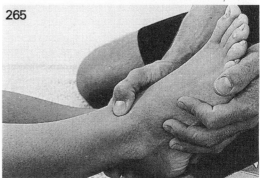

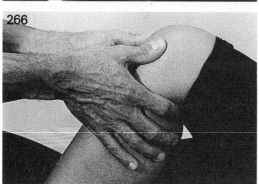

Knees
See pages 174-176 for sequence. Use St 35 (*fig. 266*) and extra points (*fig. 267*). St 36 (*fig. 268*), GB 34 (*fig. 269*), Sp 9 (*fig. 270*), Liv 8 (*fig. 271*), UB 40 (*fig. 272*).

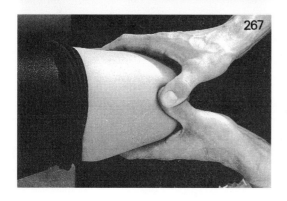

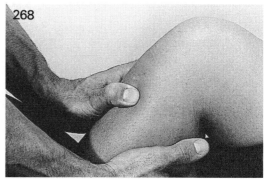

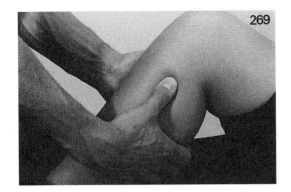

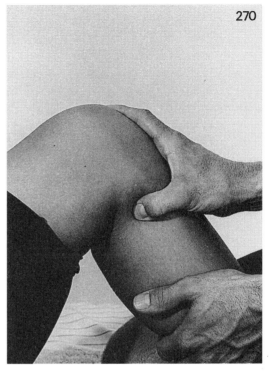

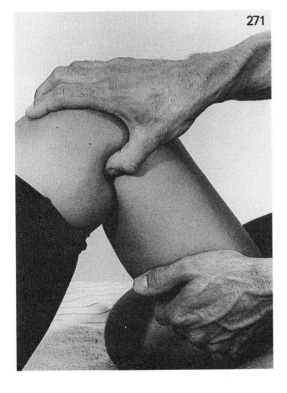

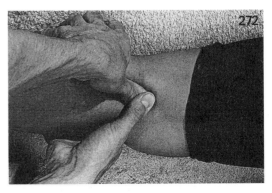

Hips and buttocks

This area can be massaged in two main positions.

a) Receiver lying on their side, with the upper leg bent at the knee in the 'recovery' position. This is especially good for getting to the joint and buttock area.

Giver kneeling with outside foot up level with receiver's hips.

1) Rotate fleshy part of buttock with hands crossed palm on back of hand *(fig. 273)*. Both ways.

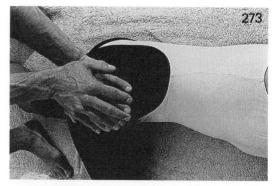

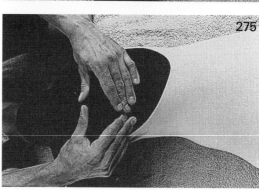

2) Effleurage *(fig. 274)*, knead, squeeze buttocks *(fig. 275)*.

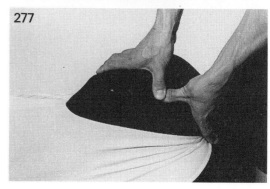

3) Thumbs pressing into buttocks in lines to cover whole buttock area. *Points:* GB 29 *(fig. 276)*, GB 30 *(fig. 277)*, UB 54 *(fig. 278)*, UB 36 *(fig. 279)*.

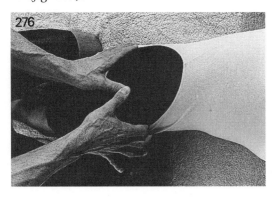

278

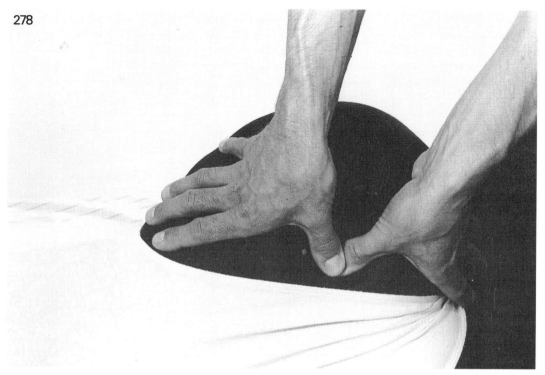

279

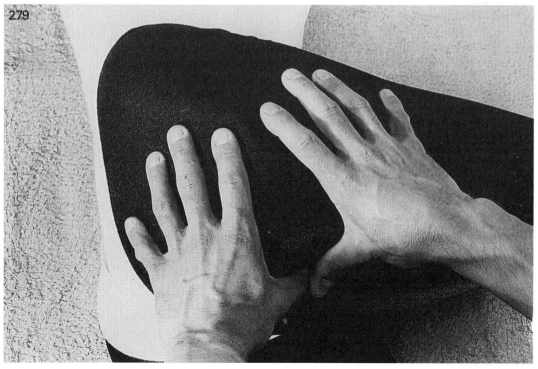

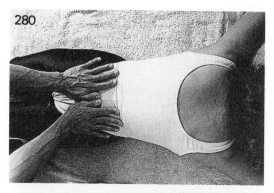

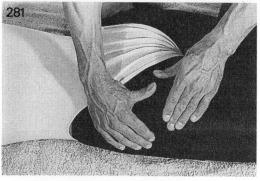

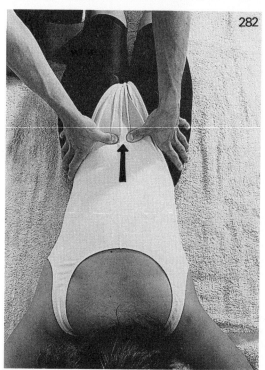

b) Receiver lying on front. This is useful for getting to the area and the buttocks, both sides at the same time. Giver's position as before.

1) Effleurage over buttocks and up lower back (*fig. 280*).

2) Kneading and squeezing the buttocks (*fig. 280*).

3) Thumbs over buttocks in lines as before, two hands separately this time. *Points:* UB 27 to 36 (*fig. 282*), and 53/54 (*fig. 283*); GB 30 (*fig. 284*).

The above sequence is appropriate for injuries to the specific areas mentioned. Where time permits, and for overall beneficial effects on the whole leg and buttock area, you can use the following sequences:

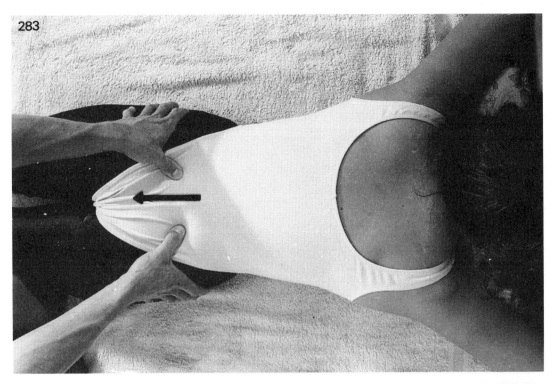

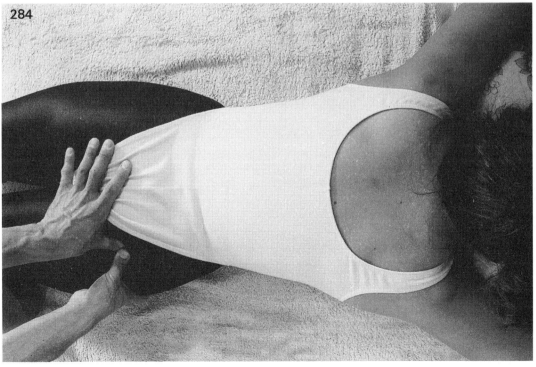

Back of legs

Note: Position of hand during effleurage on legs is slightly different from the description in Chapter 2. It should be done with hands facing across leg in opposite directions.

Cover the leg you're not working on; pad upper ankles. Kneel alongside calf. Make contact. Apply oil to hands and begin effleurage of entire leg and buttock (*figs. 285, 286 and 287*). If your partner is not comfortable having the buttocks worked on, then just work up to the top of the thigh. Be careful when leaning pressure into strokes not to lean into back of knee. To apply more pressure into back of thigh, simply move up into knees and lean more pressure into stroke. Repeat this stroke 20 times. Then lean thumb gradually into calf from ankle up to knee. Lean heels of hand into same movement (*figs. 288 and 289*). Repeat these two strokes on back of thigh, moving your position accordingly. You may use more pressure on thighs. Include the buttocks into this stroke on the thighs. Wide

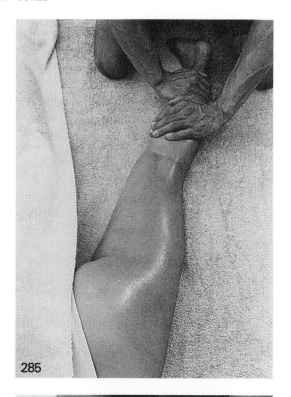

285

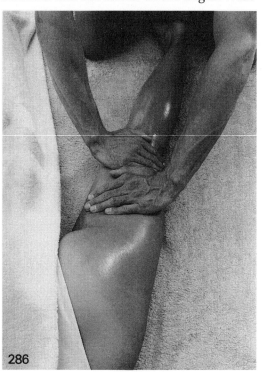

286

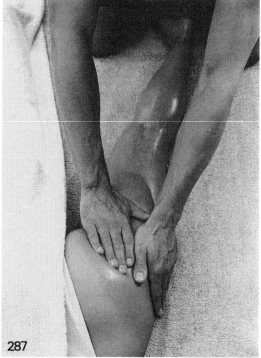

287

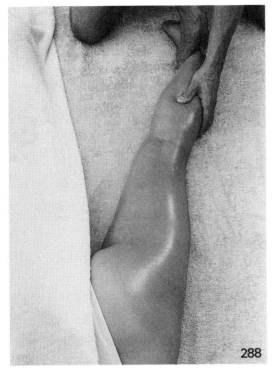

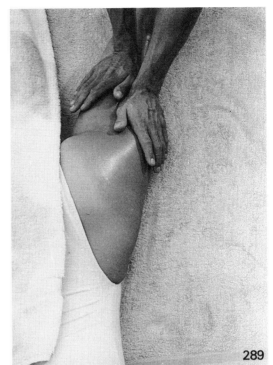

knees alongside the body. Knead, wring and pull buttocks, thighs and calves (*figs. 290, 291 and 292*). Come back to original position at feet and effleurage centre leg and buttock including foot at least 20 times. Repeat same sequence on the leg, covering leg you have just worked on.

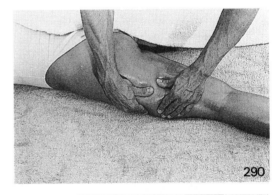

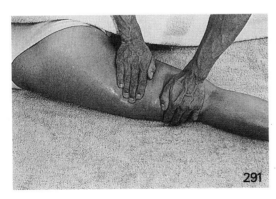

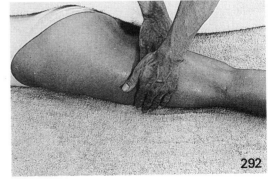

Front of legs

1) Cover both legs with a large towel or blanket.

2) Make contact with leg you're going to work on.

3) Uncover leg, apply oil to hand and begin effleurage. Allow outside hand to sweep around outside of thigh and inside hand around inside of thigh (*fig. 293*). Repeat at least 20 times.

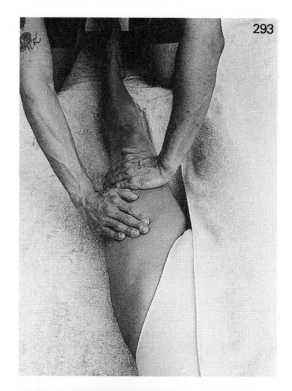

293

NB: Avoid going too high up inside of partner's thigh — it may feel invasive. Also avoid giving pressure directly to knee area.

4) Lean heels of hands into either side of shin bone and up to knee (*fig. 294*). Pull hands down again to ankle and repeat ten times.

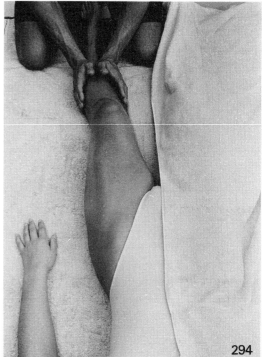

294

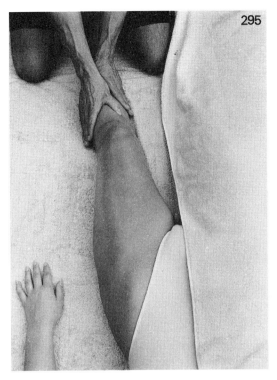

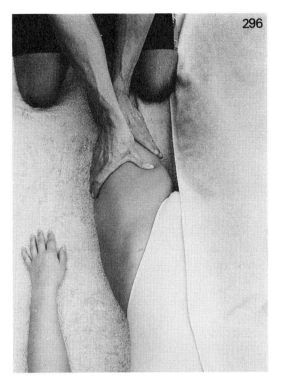

5) Lean thumbs in (crossed) either side of shin to knee (*fig. 295*). Move your position up to knee and repeat same movement on thigh (*fig. 296*).

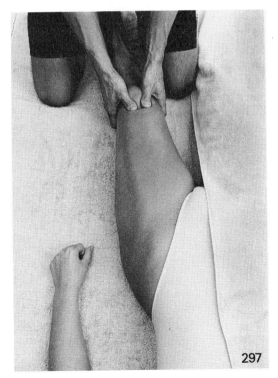

6) In between these movements you may wrap hands around knees and circle entire joint with thumbs (*fig. 297*).

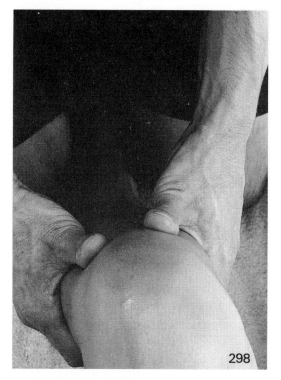

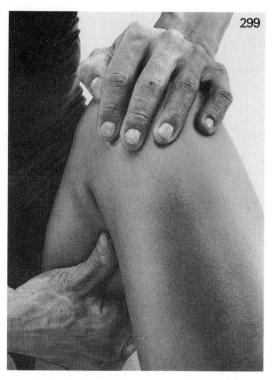

7) Bend receiver's knee at 90 degrees and bring foot flat on floor. Support the foot and ankle with both knees hugging either side, kneeling to face their head. 'Walk' down calf from behind knee to ankle using fingers like playing the piano (*fig. 298*). Lean back to increase pressure. Alternatively, support knee with one hand and lean in, squeezing and kneading calf muscle with thumb and fingers (*fig. 299*). Change hands and repeat.

8) Wide knees position: knead, wring and pull thigh. Come down to ankle again. Complete sequence with effleurage of whole leg 20 times. The foot sequence can be included at this point.

Bach flower remedies

Disliking oneself,
overeating: Crab apple

Never content with
present progress: Rock water

Obsessive, over-zealous,
over-exercising: Vervain

Despondency, losing
heart/interest in one's
progress: Gentian

Oils

Oils can be used with massage to reduce tension on a regular basis. This will reduce the risk of injury during exercise and the likelihood of muscle tension after exercise. They can also be used effectively in baths.

Baths: Relaxing, maintenance oils — Lavender, Camomile, Neroli, Ylang-ylang, Marjoram, Geranium. Stimulating maintenance oils — Rosemary, Juniper, Cypress, Grapefruit, Orange, Peppermint, Lemongrass.

Massage: Pre-exercise — See stimulating bath oils. After exercise: Marjoram, Lemongrass, Camomile, Lavender, Geranium.

Self-esteem

○ I am good enough right now.
○ I am naturally slim, and my body is returning to its correct weight.
○ It's safe for me to let go of my excess weight.
○ It's safe for me to be light and slim.
○ I am now loving my body and giving it the very best.
○ It's safe for me to feel all my feelings.
○ I accept myself completely.
○ I love and approve of myself completely.
○ My body is growing in health and vitality every day.
○ I now only ever eat when I'm hungry.
○ I now relax by exercising my body.
○ The more I exercise, the more I relax and enjoy my body.
○ My body is getting stronger and fitter every day.

To end with here is a quote from Avicenna, who was the most outstanding of Arab physicians and wrote the following advice on massage and athletes during the 10th century, when Arab medicine was the most advanced in the Western world:

There is a friction [massage] of preparation, which comes before exercise . . . then there is a friction of restoration, which comes after exercise and is called rest-inducing friction. The object of this is the resolution of superfluities retained in the muscles, not evacuated by exercise, that they may be evaporated, and that fatigue may not occur. This friction must be done smoothly and gently.

11

Conclusions

We have seen the crucial role played by touch in the healthy development of the individual. From the gentle embrace of the amniotic fluid in the womb, through the process of birth itself to the affectionate caresses of first our parents, then our partners and finally our own children. We observed the physiological effects of the touch stimulus especially on the development of the nervous system and how this affects normal growth and development. Equally, we noted the psychological importance of touch in promoting healthy self-esteem and emotional integration. In particular we distinguished the different experiences of men and women in our society with regard to touch, as well as the many and varied touch practices and taboos within different cultures. We identified too the clear role of structured touch in the form of massage both to self and to partners, family and friends. It was seen that some cultures, particularly in the East, enjoy a greater degree of acceptance of this role than our own and that the massage therapies have traditionally thrived in societies such as the Chinese, Japanese and Indian.

We noted however that a more recent trend in Western countries has been towards rediscovering the benefits of both our own massage traditions as well as those from other countries. Swedish-based muscular and deep tissue as well as intuitive massage, aromatherapy, shiatsu, acupuncture, pulsing, rolfing and reflexology — all have started to gain great popularity. As our society was previously not at all touch-conscious, this development is hardly a surprising one and performs, in fact, a very legitimate and needed function of literally putting us back 'in touch' with one another. Despite the unfortunate image of massage in recent years, people are once again looking to it as a healthy and totally natural way of improving their overall health and the way they feel about themselves. For men especially, massage offers them an opportunity to nurture and to nourish in a way that traditionally, only women have been trained to do. It affords them the chance to step out of the stereotypical role which limits their emotional and physical intimacy with others. Thus we can see massage may impact the traditional roles of men and women in society and cause a breakthrough in how we relate to one another on all levels.

Finally, we have noted a huge shift in personal and planetary awareness in our current generation. Issues which have forced their way into public consciousness in recent years have included changing attitudes towards sex and gender and the nature of relationships in general, increased concern for the environment, reflected in the Green movement and perhaps most significant of all, increased personal responsibility in the area of health and prevention of disease. Of all the health pratices which have begun to complement and in some cases even replace hitherto orthodox medicine, massage is the oldest, simplest and most natural.

It is not surprising, then, that in the age of high-tech communications, where relationships with machines are often more highly involved than these between human beings, we should be desperately trying to keep 'in touch' on a human level. One of the most concerted and substantial technological ahievements of this century to date — the placing of a man on the moon — actually produced astronauts whose lasting achievement may be to caution us against too rapid and environmentally destructive technological progress. Many of them, since the space programme, have spent time and money trying to share with us their experience of a 'common para-consciousness' which connects each part of a giant information system we call the Universe. Unless we understand that we are all inextricably linked together, our minds and bodies, our environment, even present and future in a web of shared communication and relationship, we cannot hope to experience the fullness of life itself. In its own way, massage makes a valuable contribution, not only to our immediate health and happiness, but to our deeper communion with life and its higher purpose.

Now, more than ever, is a time of intense and rapid change in the world. Within the last 100 years, a small fraction of the Earth's history, we have developed the technology to travel at huge speeds both in this world and in space, to harness vast energy sources, including the ability to destroy ourselves several times over, even to genetically engineer life itself. Yet the search for personal happiness and fulfilment persists in all of us.

We assert that, through experiencing the joys and simple pleasure of both giving and receiving bodily contact through massage, we can enrich the quality of our lives immeasurably.

Massage and peace of mind

Massage is the fastest growing of the complementary therapies. In the past few years it has gained phenomenal acceptance with the general public and the medical establishment. From being a therapy which was seen as having value really only in the realm of physiotherapy and sports injuries, it now forms part of the treatment programme for cancer and cardiac recovery patients in hospitals. This progress has been happening during the past 20 years but has speeded up enormously in the past two or three years. Huge numbers of nurses and physiotherapists are taking massage courses themselves and incorporating their new skill in their hospital routines. Nurses in particular have tremendous scope for including massage as a treatment following the development of 'primary care' nursing where nurses are appointed to a particular patient for the duration of the hospital stay. A number of leading teaching hospitals in Britain are now including the practice of massage within nursing training. One of the great advantages of massage above all other forms of treatment is that it is a healing art and practical skill that is accessible to everyone. We all have the instinctive ability to help another through our caring touch. Not only can we bring great tangible benefits to others, but we, as the givers, also gain enormously through the gift of giving. The stroking of animals is known to lower blood pressure and promote relaxation in the giver; this aptly demonstrates our inherent human need to both give and receive care and affection to our fellow human beings and also the animal and plant kingdoms.

Illness and well-being are directly connected to both the physical expression of love to others and to the receiving of love for ourselves. Massage provides the unequalled opportunity to touch and be touched on a level that words and kind thoughts could never reach. Massage really is an extraordinary panacea for the excesses of our modern civilization. In the obsessively materialistic West, we are all seeking ways of repairing and maintaining our health and energy levels: and seeking for that ever elusive 'peace of mind'. So much of our life revolves around finding ways of securing peace of mind, usually focused on bigger home, a better-paid job and secure retirement. Peace of mind is a state that can only ever be generated from within, regardless, to a large extent, of our external circumstances.

Peace of mind comes from physical relaxation and mental calm. Many of us may never actually have fully experienced either of these qualities and attaining them alone may be extremely difficult. We have simply lost the ability to relax. Massage from a caring therapist or friend will gently and effortlessly return us to a natural way of being where we experience 'peace of mind' as a tangible physical feeling and a deep sense of peace and well-being. It is in returning to this natural state of internal harmony and ease that we gain inner calm and tranquillity. Our external world may be full of turmoil and fear, but in taking control of our internal world and resonating calm and tranquillity, we begin to affect and impact that outside world. We all have our part to play in affecting both our immediate environment and the world at large. By taking responsibility for your peace and contributing to others, you make a difference in the lives of all those around you and in effect the entire planet.

When we operate from fear and anxiety, we create a dangerous world full of fear and anxiety. It is within our individual power to operate out of love, trust and internal tranquillity. What a totally different world we could then create. Indeed, we are already moving into a very important age which is quite unlike the fear-filled 70s and 80s. The superpower leaders are beginning to trust and communicate and for two cultures locked in 'cold war' for over 40 years, this is outstanding progress towards world peace. Of course much remains to be done but it is only when we, as individuals, take total responsibility for creating our own peace and extending it out that real, permanent universal peace and happiness can be attained.

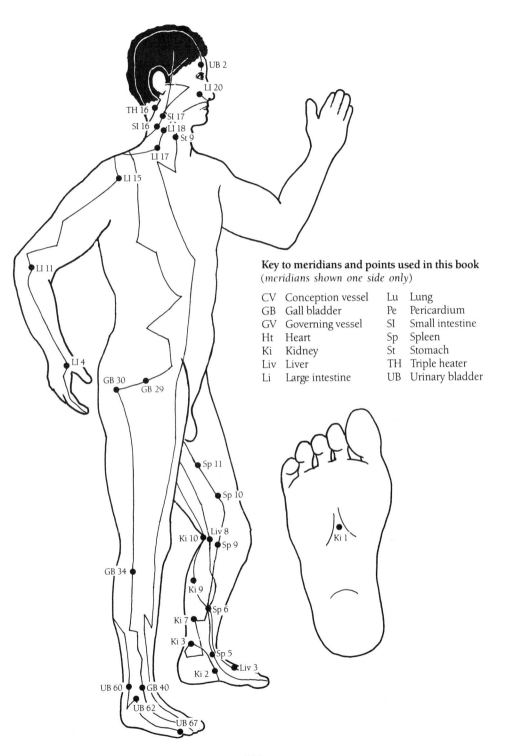

Key to meridians and points used in this book
(*meridians shown one side only*)

CV	Conception vessel	Lu	Lung
GB	Gall bladder	Pe	Pericardium
GV	Governing vessel	SI	Small intestine
Ht	Heart	Sp	Spleen
Ki	Kidney	St	Stomach
Liv	Liver	TH	Triple heater
Li	Large intestine	UB	Urinary bladder

181

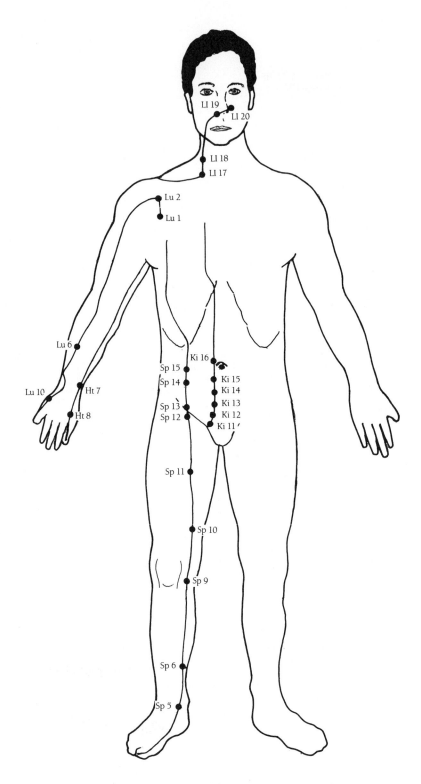

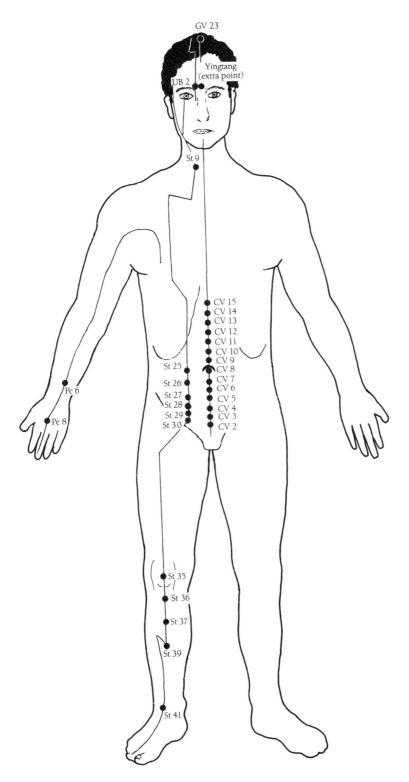

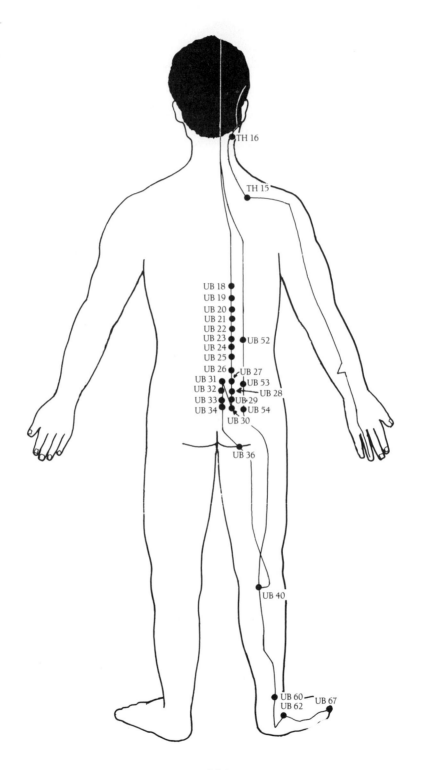

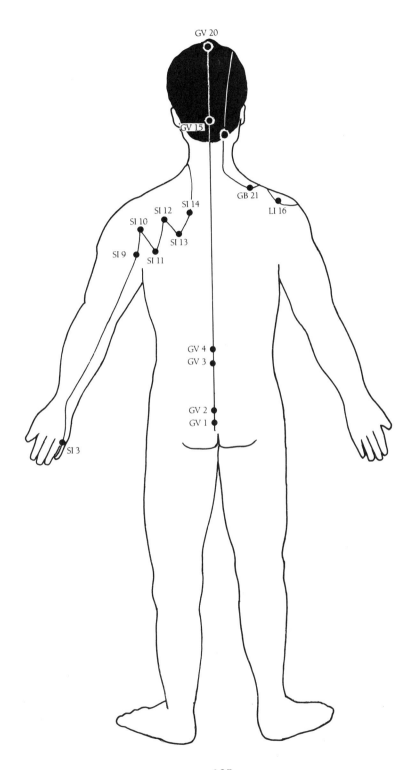

Bibliography

Shiatsu

Zen Imagery Exercises Shizuto Masunaga (Japan Publications)

Zen Shiatsu Shizuto Masunaga (Japan Publications)

Tsubo — Vital Points for Oriental Therapy Katsusuke Serizawa (Japan Publications)

Book of Do-In Michio Kushi (Japan Publications)

Shiatsu Therapy Toru Namikoshi (Japan Publications)

Barefoot Shiatsu Shizuko Yamamoto (Japan Publications)

Do It Yourself Shiatsu Wataru Ohashi (Unwin Hyman)

The Shiatsu Way to Health Toru Namikoshi (Kodansha Int. Ltd.)

Shiatsu Practitioner's Manual Saul Goodman (Infitech Pub.)

Natural Healing through Macrobiotics Michio Kushi (Japan Publications)

The Way to Locate Acu-Points edited by Yang Jiasan (Foreign Lang. Press)

Massage

The Book of Massage Clare Maxwell-Hudson (Ebury Press)

Touching Ashley Montagu (Harper and Row)

The Complete Book of Swedish Massage Armand Maanum (Harper and Row)

Massage for Common Ailments Sarah Thomas (Sidgwick and Jackson)

Massage and Loving Anne Hooper (Unwin Hyman)

The Complete Book of Massage Clare Maxwell-Hudson (Dorling Kindersley)

The Magic of Massage Ouida West (Century)

Massage (Time-Life Books)

The Bodywork Book Nevill Drury (Prism Press)

Massage and Peaceful Pregnancy Gordon Inkeles (Unwin Paperbacks)

Massage for Healing and Relaxation Carola Beresford-Cooke (Arlington Books)

Super Massage Gordon Inkeles (Piatkus)

Massage Ken Eyerman (Sidgwick and Jackson)

Massage Therapy Richard Jackson (Thorsons)

Baby Massage Peter Walker (Bloomsbury)

The Massage Book George Downing (Penguin)

Aromatherapy

Aromatherapy Judith Jackson (Dorling Kindersley)

Aromatherapy — An A-Z Patricia Davis (C.W. Daniel Co. Ltd)

Bach flower remedies

Bach Flower Therapy Mechthild Scheffer (Thorsons)

Flower Remedies to the Rescue Gregory Vlamis (Thorsons)

Self-esteem

You Can Heal Your Life Louise L. Hay (Eden Grove Edns)

Matthew Manning's Guide to Self-healing Matthew Manning (Thorsons)

I Deserve Love Sondra Ray (Celestial Arts)

Loving Relationships Sondra Ray (Celestial Arts)

Creative Visualization Shakti Gawain (Bantam)

Living in the Light Shakti Gawain (Eden Grove)

Love is Letting Go of Fear Gerald Jampolsky (Celestial Arts)

Miscellaneous

Black's Medical Dictionary William A. R. Thomson (A. & C. Black)

Stress without Distress Hans Selye (Signet)

The Yellow Emperor's Classic of Internal Medicine Trans. by Ilza Veith (University of California Press)

The Canon of Acupuncture Kisunu & Yunkyo Lee (Hong Sung Ent. Ltd)

Iron Shirt Chi Kung. Vol 1 Mantak Chia (Healing Tao Books)

Chinese Qi Gong Therapy Zhang Mingwu & Son Xingyuan (Shandong Science and Technology Press)

Taoist Ways to Transform Stress into Vitality Mantak Chia (Healing Tao Press)

Awaken Healing Energy through the Tao Mantak Chia (Aurora Press)

Taoist Secrets of Love — Cultivating Male Sexual Energy Mantak Chia (Aurora Press)

Taoist Secrets of Love — Cultivating Female Sexual Energy Mantak Chia (Aurora Press)

Acupressure, Yoga and You Louise Taylor and Betty Bryant (Japan Publications)

Yoga and Pregnancy Sophie Hoare (Unwin Paperbacks)

New Active Birth Janet Balaskas (Unwin Paperbacks)

Wise Woman Herbal for the Childbearing Year Susun S. Weed (Ashtree Publishing)

Female Cycles Paula Weideger (Women's Press)

Neal's Yard Natural Remedies (Arkana)

The Wright Diet Celia Wright (Grafton)

Index

Figures in italics refer to illustrations